Early Modern History: Society and Culture

This series encompasses European topics in the areas of social, political and cultural history from 1400 to 1800. It will also include colonial subjects where the themes and methodologies have direct relevance to, and influence on, European history.

More information about this series at
http://www.springer.com/series/15033

Daphna Oren-Magidor

Infertility in Early Modern England

palgrave
macmillan

Daphna Oren-Magidor
Buber Society of Fellows
Hebrew University of Jerusalem
Jerusalem, Israel

Early Modern History: Society and Culture
ISBN 978-1-137-47667-8 ISBN 978-1-137-47668-5 (eBook)
DOI 10.1057/978-1-137-47668-5

Library of Congress Control Number: 2017943392

Printed on acid-free paper

This Palgrave Macmillan imprint is published by Springer Nature
The registered company is Macmillan Publishers Ltd.
The registered company address is: The Campus, 4 Crinan Street, London, N1 9XW, United Kingdom

To my parents, Sarah and Menachem, for giving me everything I needed to get here.

Acknowledgements

In the course of writing this book, I've accrued many debts. First, my deepest thanks are owed to those institutions whose generous funding has enabled me to conduct my research: the graduate school at Brown University, the Mellon-CLIR Fellowship for Dissertation Research in Original Sources, the George L. Mosse Postdoctoral Fellowship in the History of Gender and Sexuality at the Hebrew University, and most recently the Martin Buber Society of Fellows in the Humanities and Social Sciences. I would also like to thank the staffs of libraries and reading rooms all over the United Kingdom and beyond, especially those of the British Library and of Princeton's Rare Books and Manuscripts department. I would also like to thank the trustees of the British Museum and the Pepys Library, Magdalene College, Cambridge, for permission to publish the images in this book.

I was fortunate to have two wonderful scholarly homes during the writing of this book. The colleagues, teachers and mentors at Brown University who have made an indelible mark on my work and my life are too numerous to mention, but I would like to thank all of those who made my years in Providence so meaningful. Above all, Tim Harris has been a dedicated advisor, whose support of this project has been crucial in bringing it completion, and Tara Nummedal's input, advice and mentorship have been invaluable, and I am deeply grateful to both of them. Adam and Marina Darlow's presence in Providence made our life there that much sweeter.

I am grateful to all of my colleagues and friends in the Buber Fellows for providing a stimulating and supportive intellectual environment, and in particular to Yael Baron, Ruth HaCohen and Verena Krebs. Dror Wahrman, Moshe Sluhovsky and Aya Elyada were instrumental in making me feel welcome in the department of History in Jerusalem. Moshe has also supported me in this endeavour from the moment the idea was merely a glint in a doctoral candidate's eye until the last draft of the book, and I cannot thank him enough for his constant mentorship and guidance.

Kelly Feinstein-Johnson has read innumerable drafts of this work and has been generous with her astute advice. More importantly, her friendship has been a true gift in my life. Thanks also to the anonymous readers who reviewed the manuscript and offered excellent advice, as well as the many other people who have read portions of this text throughout its creation. Any errors that remain are entirely my own.

I would not be typing these words today if it were not for my family. My father, Menachem, is a mathematician with a historian's heart. Whatever love I have of history, I first learned it from him. My mother, Sarah, has read and edited more versions of this research than can be counted, and has contributed superb insights from her own professional experience of fertility treatments. My love and thanks go to both of them, and also to my three sisters, who have each, in their own way, given something to this study.

Finally, these few lines will never be enough to thank Hanan Oren for being my partner in everything, so I will just say wava, ding. You know what that means.

Contents

A Note for Readers

All spelling has been maintained in its original form, with additions or explanations appearing in square brackets. Original punctuation has largely been preserved, but occasionally some punctuation has been added where it was crucial for understanding. All dates have been preserved as in the original sources.

Abbreviations

Add.	Additional Manuscripts
BL	British Library
Bodl.	Bodleian Library
CCRO	Cheshire and Chester Record Office
CSPVen	Calendar of State Papers, Venetian
FSL	Folger Shakespeare Library
KHLC	Kent History and Library Centre
KJV	The Bible, King James Version
WL	Wellcome Library
WSRO	West Sussex Record Office

List of Figures

CHAPTER 1

Introduction

Mary Whitelocke wanted to make sure that her son Samuel knew that he was special, a child given to her by God after she had suffered through many years of childlessness. As Samuel was entering manhood in the 1660s, Mary wrote a spiritual memoir of her life, intending to educate her son about his birth and advise him how to conduct his life. In the process, Whitelocke created an unparalleled and often heart-wrenching account of an early modern woman's experience of infertility. Mary described her first married years thus: 'Though I had as much outward comforts as this world could afford, yet I did thinke offen: Lord what is all this to me seeing I goe childless.' Despite her love for her first husband and the happiness of her marriage, Mary wrote that she 'did very offen greif and morne for the want of children in this life'.[1] Samuel was the first of several children born to Mary and her second husband, Bulstrode Whitelocke. Although she was far from childless when she wrote the memoir, it retains the raw emotion engendered by the fourteen childless years of her first marriage. The pain and difficulty of being a childless married woman had a powerful hold on Whitelocke long after she had become a mother. Bulstrode had ten children from two previous marriages when he married Mary in 1650, and had no need for heirs. This did not mitigate Mary's desire for a child. Like many women of her time, she wanted a child of her own.

D. Oren-Magidor, *Infertility in Early Modern England*,
Early Modern History: Society and Culture,
DOI 10.1057/978-1-137-47668-5_1

Infertility in Early Modern England examines fertility problems both as medical conditions and as social issues. It argues that infertility was not solely a personal misfortune, but was rather a source of social and cultural anxiety. The centrality of childbearing to the early modern social order meant that the idea of failed reproduction was destabilizing. Therefore, early modern couples who did not conceive shortly after marriage faced considerable pressure from family and friends, and were routinely questioned about their reproductive plans. Moreover, although there is only limited evidence of infertile people being actively mocked for their condition, early modern culture was replete with negative portrayals of infertility, defining infertile men as emasculated and infertile women as immoral and transgressive of gendered boundaries. These views were connected to the religious meaning of reproduction in this period, which was seen as nothing short of women's avenue to salvation. Therefore, a woman who did not conceive was suspected of being sinful. Indeed, this study elucidates the crucial significance of religion to every aspect of the experience of infertility in this period. Devout men and women were encouraged to understand their childlessness as either a punishment for sins or a test of faith designed by divine providence to teach them a lesson in humility and acceptance. They were told to pray earnestly for children, but also to accept that if their prayers were not answered, this was because there was some deeper meaning to their infertility. They were therefore encouraged to consider childlessness as a chance to place their efforts on good works, charity and piety. But the impact of religion was not merely overt, nor limited to the texts of sermons or religious guidebooks. Instead, religion also underlay medical explanations of infertility. Rather than being morally neutral, medical texts instead argued that sterility was caused by behavioural factors which were closely linked to sin: promiscuity, lust, gluttony, idleness and wrath. The treatment of fertility problems was also linked to religion, as the efficacy of medical treatment was understood as a God-given gift, and patients were advised to practice specific forms of prayer before taking some treatments. It is not surprising that religion played an important role in the management of a medical condition in this period, but the important social and cultural nature of fertility problems highlights the precise ways in which early modern patients gave meaning to their suffering through faith, found comfort in religious practice and ritual, and linked their views of the body and its illness with their views of morality and salvation.

Some scholars have downplayed the significance of infertility in early modern English society. Alan Macfarlane argues that, while early modern couples wanted children for a variety of practical and emotional reasons, it was not a 'tragedy' if they could not have any.[2] A more recent survey of gender relations in this period states simply that while infertility was a part of many families' lives, 'fertility does not seem to have been used as a measure of masculinity or femininity'.[3] It is true that early modern men and women were not judged on their ability to produce as many children as possible. Indeed, as Macfarlane points out, over-large families were criticized.[4] However, this dismissal of the significance of infertility does not fully take into account the personal emotional impact of infertility on married couples. This impact was not only the result of practical concerns such as providing heirs or working hands, nor of an abstract 'desire for children'. Rather, infertility sat at the centre of a web that tied together a providential religious outlook that saw illness and health, fertility and infertility as directly ordained by God, with a highly gendered social order that had the nuclear family as its foundation.[5] This book will highlight the complicated ways in which early modern beliefs about the infertile body worked together with a religious world view that connected fertility to salvation and infertility to sin, and how these in turn fitted into a social order that encouraged dominant, self-controlled husbands and dutiful, chaste, obedient wives. Infertility distanced couples, and especially women, from the early modern ideals of body, faith and family, and in doing so it highlighted extant anxieties about society and gender, masculinity and femininity.[6]

Motherhood was central to women's identity in early modern England.[7] Certainly, not all women married, let alone bore children, but the ideology of the period highlighted marriage and motherhood as the ideal state for women.[8] House, family and children were the role that women were allotted by divine providence.[9] Childbearing was routinely described as the primary purpose of marriage, although not the only one.[10] The role of childbearing in maintaining the social order has been well established by scholars such as Patricia Crawford, Linda Pollock and Laura Gowing.[11] They have also highlighted the birthing chamber as a space for homosocial support on the one hand and for policing of women on the other, as women examined each other's bodies for signs of illicit pregnancy or exchanged gossip and rumours.[12] Scholars have also documented the disruptive role of extramarital childbearing to the early modern social order, and early modern women's attempts to limit or prevent fertility through contraception, abortion and infanticide.[13] The impact of non-normative reproduction has been studied at length, but scholars have shown more interest in attempts to uncover hidden births outside marriage, than failed births within its confines. Yet, as Lisa Smith points out, 'unlike illegitimate births, sterility was a medical problem that happened within the context of legitimate sexuality and reproduction and emphasises the existence of women's bodies within the public domain. A woman's failure to become pregnant and her attempts to cure her sterility were publicly witnessed and discussed.'[14]

Despite the significance of fertility problems, the study of infertility has been somewhat of a footnote in the growing historiography on reproduction, receiving only limited attention until recently. Angus McLaren devoted one chapter of his book on reproduction to infertility, the rest dealing with attempts to limit fertility rather than promote it.[15] Crawford, Sara Mendelson, Antonia Fraser and others have devoted a few words or paragraphs to infertility in larger studies of the role of women in early modern society.[16] Only in the past decade or so has there been a more concerted effort to study the history of early modern infertility, primarily by historians of medicine who have offered in-depth analyses of reproductive difficulties as medical conditions and have placed it within the broader context of a social history of medicine.[17] Jennifer Evans has studied the use of aphrodisiacs to treat fertility problems stemming from sexual dysfunction, and has also written several articles on medical aspects of fertility treatments.[18] Sarah Toulalan has expanded the limits of discussions of fertility by asking how old age was related to reproduction in this period, and has also considered beliefs about fatness and fertility.[19] Helen Berry and Elizabeth Foyster have offered an illuminating examination of male childlessness in this period, with a social rather than a medical focus, adding an important reminder that infertility was not only a 'woman's problem'.[20] This book builds on the existing scholarship, but offers a more well-rounded view of fertility problems in their medical and sociocultural dimensions.

Although the exact prevalence of early modern infertility is difficult to assess, many couples did encounter fertility problems during their lives. Naomi Tadmor argues that approximately one in five English marriages were childless.[21] According to one historical demographic study of English families, approximately 7–10 per cent of marriages between 1540 and 1750 in which both husband and wife were single at marriage and the wife lived to be fifty had no children. Given the lack of reliable contraception, and the unlikelihood that most of these marriages were celibate, this strongly suggests that either the husband or the wife (or both) were infertile.[22] For marriages that lasted at least ten years, but not until the wife was fifty, the study found that about 6 per cent of those married between the ages of twenty and twenty-four and 8 per cent of those married between twenty-five and twenty-nine did not have children for at least ten years after marriage, again strongly suggesting a fertility problem.[23] Another demographic study collected data from sixteen English parishes between 1550 and 1849, and found that approximately 4.6 per cent of women who got married between the ages of twenty and twenty-four never gave birth to a living child after their marriage, and this percentage goes up to 9.1 per cent for women who married between the ages of twenty-five and twenty-nine.[24] These data do not give an aggregate picture of the total number of early modern couples who were infertile, but they do demonstrate that infertility was not a minor or insignificant problem. As Laura Gowing states succinctly, 'many marriages were childless'.[25]

These numbers are only part of the picture. Many people suffered from fertility problems but did not remain childless throughout their lives. Some of the subjects of this book went through a period of infertility at the beginning of their marriages, with the attendant emotional difficulties and medical treatment, before successfully giving birth to one or more children. In other cases, such as that of Mary Whitelocke, a man or a woman might be childless during a first marriage, only to discover that they had no difficulty having children with a second spouse. Moreover, some of the subjects in this book did not suffer from primary infertility, meaning an inability to have children at all, but rather from secondary infertility, meaning that they did had one child and then faced difficulties when they wanted to have additional children. Such couples would not make their way into statistics of childless marriages, but this did not mean that they did not worry about their fertility problems or seek to treat them.

The modern term 'fertility problems' used here includes the inability to conceive, which is the most commonplace meaning of 'infertility' but is not limited to it. Fertility problems could also be recurring miscarriages and stillbirths, as well as recurring premature labours resulting in the inevitable death of the infant within hours of birth. In other words, this book does not focus only a narrow definition of 'infertility' as an inability to conceive, but on a broad definition of 'infertility' or 'fertility problems' as any condition that hindered a couple from having viable children who could survive outside the womb. The book thus has room for women such as Elizabeth Pepys, who had no children and was likely never pregnant (probably because of her husband Samuel's medical condition rather than her own).[26] It also has room for women such as Queen Anne, who was pregnant seventeen times in her life, yet had only three children who survived beyond the first hours of life and was childless at the end of her fertile years. Anne had no difficulty conceiving, but her recurring miscarriages, stillbirths and premature births, as well as her irregular menstruation, place her firmly within the category of people suffering from fertility problems in the early modern period, and thus well within the scope of this study. That she actively sought treatment for those conditions only makes this clearer.[27] Men will also appear in this book, both because they suffered from fertility problems themselves and because they sought treatments for their wives' infertility. However, while early modern medicine recognized the existence of male infertility, in practice women were usually 'blamed' for childlessness and treated for it. Therefore, the 'typical' fertility patient was a woman, and some sections of the book will deal almost exclusively with women.

Chronologically, this study begins in about 1540, when the first in a long series of popular midwifery manuals in English was published.[28] This allowed for a wider dissemination of formal medical knowledge about conception and pregnancy. The period that followed was also one in which the Reformation took hold in England, and with it religious and social tumult. While there was much continuity between Catholic and Protestant England, and many ideas about gender and sexuality circulated throughout all of Europe in this period, the Reformed theology did more to highlight childbearing as the main avenue for female piety. Catholic women had, at least in theory, two avenues for performing their religious duty: the more common avenue of marriage and childbirth, and the 'sacred' avenue of virginity.[29] By contrast, Protestantism highlighted marriage as 'the best Christian life' and objected to celibacy as impractical for most. Martin Luther preached that 'although women had brought about the Fall, they were sanctified by the bearing of children', and this idea was echoed by other reformers.[30] For Protestant women, therefore, reproduction was a central avenue towards the fulfilment of their religious duties. The Reformation also irrevocably altered therapeutic practices, by eroding a rich tapestry of rituals pertaining to saintly intervention in medical problems.[31] Women were now encouraged to pray to God alone and put their trust in divine providence. Providence was central to early modern people's understanding of infertility. They saw childlessness as either a test of faith or a punishment of sins, and the cure of infertility as an act of God. While this view was particularly powerful within the godly or 'Puritan' milieu to which women like Mary Whitelocke belonged, Alexandra Walsham demonstrates that it was prevalent in all forms of English Christianity in the sixteenth and seventeenth centuries.[32] By the eighteenth century, this providential world view was on the wane. The eighteenth century also saw a significant change in the practice of women's medicine. As male midwives gained prominence, they also sought to carve themselves a place of recognition as physicians, rather than only obstetric technicians. Physicians had been showing a greater interest in women's medicine from the sixteenth century and even earlier.[33] However, from the 1720s medical schools in Britain began offering specific training courses in women's health and midwifery for male midwives, while physicians in general were developing new theoretical perspectives about gynaecology.[34]

There is no strict cut-off point for the transition away from providential Christianity or into a new kind of women's medicine, and many of the practices and perceptions of infertility presented in this book continued well into the eighteenth century. Nonetheless, the period around the end of Queen Anne's reign in 1714 marks a convenient end point for this study, as Anne was the last in a long line of English monarchs who suffered from fertility problems. Because of the public and political nature of royal childbearing, royal infertility was often better documented than more private cases, so that many of the examples in this book will draw on the stories of royal or aristocratic women. Where possible the book will rely on more ordinary people, notably Mary Whitelocke, who was the daughter of a wealthy London grocer, but also other women and men who wrote letters, diaries, poems and memoirs describing different aspects of infertility. A somewhat disproportionate number of these can be described as 'godly' or Puritan, because this milieu encouraged women, in particular, to write spiritual diaries and keep a record of their lives and their prayers, but members of other religious and social groups will appear.[35] Largely, however, this book will be limited to a discussion of the literate classes of early modern society. Glimpses of how the illiterate majority experienced infertility will appear through examinations of ballad literature, defamation cases and other more 'popular' sources, but they cannot make up a complete picture of how infertility affected those in the lower classes.

Gowing points out that gender relations did not undergo any great change within the early modern period.[36] The same can also be stated regarding the experiences of infertile couples and the cultural understandings and social perceptions of infertility. Broadly speaking, there was no dramatic shift in how infertility was understood, treated or experienced between 1540 and 1714. Therefore, the chapters of this book are arranged thematically rather than chronologically, discussing different aspects of fertility problems, rather than changes over time during this period. Chapter 2 explores the personal experiences of infertile couples in this period, looking at the desire for children, the disappointment when there were no children, the response to miscarriages and the ways in which childless women, in particular, sought alternative meanings to their lives by informally adopting children, focusing on religion or seeking other methods to perpetuate themselves. It will look at personal accounts of infertility, from Mary Whitelocke's uniquely detailed memoir to less expansive but nonetheless revealing sources that demonstrate how early modern people understood infertility and lived through it. Chapter 3 examines the explanatory models for fertility problems in this period, highlighting the crucial role that religious beliefs and social norms played not only in overt claims that infertility was a punishment of sins or a test of faith, but also in the medical perceptions of infertility. By prescribing how men and women should behave in order for their bodies to be fertile, medical guidebooks inscribed religious ideology onto the body and gave it a more basic and fundamental power. Chapter 4 moves into the social sphere, looking at the social and cultural perception of infertility and of infertile people in the early modern period. Although individual infertile people were not usually targeted for overt mockery (with some exceptions), the social attitude towards infertility was very negative. Not only did religious and medical texts imply that infertile people were immoral, but cultural portrayals of infertile men and women highlighted anxieties about the social order embodied in the failure of couples to properly reproduce. These anxieties emerged in the form of a recurring trope that presented infertile women as promiscuous, domineering and adulterous, and their husbands as emasculated cuckolds. Finally, Chapter 5 looks at the methods of treating infertility, starting with the reliance on prayer and religious ritual and the belief that God played a role in both causing and curing fertility problems, and continuing to an exploration of the available medical treatments: 'kitchen physic' made at home, cures purchased from medical practitioners and 'taking the waters' at a variety of spas and baths. Together, these chapters present infertility as a medical problem that lay at the crossroads of social anxieties about gender, religious beliefs about divine providence and the proper roles of men and women, practical familial considerations and the deeply personal, deeply emotional attachment of parents to their children.

Notes

1. Mary Whitelocke, *Advice for Her Son Samuel*, Princeton University RTC01 Ms. 226. This memoir was believed lost until recently, and was known only through brief sections quoted in R.H. Whitelocke, *Memoirs, Biographical and Historical of Bulstrode Whitelocke, Lord Commissioner of the Great Seal* (London: Routledge, Warne, and Routledge, 1860). However, it re-emerged in a Sotheby's sale on December 2015 and was acquired by Princeton University. The pages in the manuscript have not been numbered as of April 2016.
2. Alan Macfarlane, *Marriage and Love in England: Modes of Reproduction 1300–1840* (Oxford: Blackwell, 1986), pp. 57–61. Helen Berry and Elizabeth A. Foyster, 'Childless Men in Early Modern England', in *The Family in Early Modern England*, ed. Helen Berry and Elizabeth A. Foyster (Cambridge: Cambridge University Press, 2007), p. 164.
3. Laura Gowing, *Gender Relations in Early Modern England* (Harlow: Pearson Education, 2012), p. 22.
4. Macfarlane, *Marriage and Love in England*, pp. 60–61.
5. Alexandra Walsham, *Providence in Early Modern England* (Oxford: Oxford University Press, 1999). Berry and Foyster, 'Childless Men in Early Modern England', pp. 165–166. Susan Dwyer Amussen, *An Ordered Society: Gender and Class in Early Modern England* (New York: Blackwell, 1988).
6. Mark Breitenberg, *Anxious Masculinity in Early Modern England* (Cambridge: Cambridge University Press, 1996), pp. 2–5. Gowing, *Gender Relations in Early Modern England*, p. 5.
7. Patricia Crawford, *Blood, Bodies, and Families in Early Modern England* (Harlow, England: Pearson/Longman, 2004), p. 179. Linda A. Pollock, 'Childbearing and Female Bonding in Early Modern England', *Social History* 22, no. 3 (1997): 287–288. Olwen H. Hufton, *The Prospect Before Her: A History of Women in Western Europe* (New York: Alfred Knopf, 1996), pp. 177–178. Berry and Foyster, 'Childless Men in Early Modern England', p. 179.
8. Sara Heller Mendelson and Patricia Crawford, *Women in Early Modern England:1550–1720* (Oxford: Oxford University Press, 1998), p. 67. On unmarried people and family relations, see Naomi Tadmor, 'Early Modern English Kinship in the Long Run: Reflections on Continuity and Change', *Continuity and Change* 25, no. 01 (2010): 15–48.

9. George Savile, *The Lady's New-Years Gift, or, Advice to a Daughter* (London: Printed by Randal Taylor, 1688), pp. 68–69.
10. Crawford, *Blood, Bodies, and Families in Early Modern England*, pp. 79–112.
11. Crawford, *Blood, Bodies, and Families in Early Modern England.* Pollock, 'Childbearing and Female Bonding in Early Modern England'. Laura Gowing, 'Secret Births and Infanticide in Seventeenth-Century England', *Past & Present*, no. 156 (1997): 87–115.
12. Gowing, 'Secret Births and Infanticide in Seventeenth-Century England'. Adrian Wilson, *The Making of Man-Midwifery: Childbirth in England, 1660–1770* (Cambridge, MA: Harvard University Press, 1995).
13. Laura Gowing, *Common Bodies: Women, Touch and Power in Seventeenth-Century England* (New Haven, CT: Yale University Press, 2003). David Cressy, *Birth, Marriage, and Death: Ritual, Religion, and the Life-Cycle in Tudor and Stuart England* (Oxford: Oxford University Press, 1997). Angus McLaren, *A History of Contraception: From Antiquity to the Present Day* (Oxford: Blackwell, 1990). Lyndal Roper, *Oedipus and the Devil: Witchcraft, Sexuality, and Religion in Early Modern Europe* (London; New York: Routledge, 1994). Alan Macfarlane, 'Illegitimacy and Illegitimates in English History', in *Bastardy and Its Comparative History: Studies in the History of Illegitimacy and Marital Nonconformism in Britain, France, Germany, Sweden, North America, Jamaica, and Japan*, ed. Peter Laslett, Karla Oosterveen and Richard Michael Smith (Cambridge, MA: Harvard University Press, 1980).
14. Lisa W. Smith, 'La Raillerie Des Femmes? Les Femmes, La Stérilité Et La Société En France a L'époque Moderne', in *Femmes En Fleurs, Femmes En Corps: Sang, Santé, Sexualités Du Moyen Age Aux Lumières*, ed. Cathy McClive and Nicole Pellegrin (Saint-Étienne: Publications de l'Université de Saint-Étienne, 2010), pp. 203–220. English translation provided by Smith at https://www.academia.edu/1021799/_La_Raillerie_des_Femmes_Les_Femmes_La_Sterilit%C3%A9_et_la_Soci%C3%A9t%C3%A9_en_France_%C3%A0_l_%C3%89poque_Moderne_.
15. Angus McLaren, *Reproductive Rituals: The Perception of Fertility in England from the Sixteenth to the Nineteenth Century* (London: Methuen, 1984).
16. Mendelson and Crawford, *Women in Early Modern England: 1550-–1720*, pp. 149–150. Antonia Fraser, *The Weaker Vessel* (New York: Knopf, 1984), pp. 62–63. Gowing, *Common Bodies*, p. 114.
17. For a survey of the current state of research on infertility see also: Daphna Oren-Magidor and Catherine Rider, 'Introduction: Infertility in Medieval and Early Modern Medicine', *Social History of Medicine* 29, no. 2 (2016): 211–223.

18. Jennifer Evans, *Aphrodisiacs, Fertility and Medicine in Early Modern England* (London: Royal Historical Society, 2014). Jennifer Evans, '"Gentle Purges Corrected with Hot Spices, Whether They Work or Not, Do Vehemently Provoke Venery": Menstrual Provocation and Procreation in Early Modern England', *Social History of Medicine* 25, no. 1 (2011): 2–19.
19. Sarah Toulalan, '"Elderly Years Cause a Total Dispaire of Conception": Old Age, Sex and Infertility in Early Modern England', *Social History of Medicine* 29, no. 2 (2015): 333–359. Sarah Toulalan, '"To[O] Much Eating Stifles the Child": Fat Bodies and Reproduction in Early Modern England', *Historical Research* 87, no. 235 (2014): 65–93.
20. Berry and Foyster, 'Childless Men in Early Modern England', pp. 158–183.
21. Tadmor, 'Early Modern English Kinship in the Long Run', 20.
22. E.A. Wrigley et al., *English Population History from Family Reconstitution 1580–1837* (Cambridge: Cambridge University Press, 1997), p. 384.
23. Wrigley et al., *English Population History from Family Reconstitution*, p. 411.
24. J. Trussell and C. Wilson, 'Sterility in a Population with Natural Fertility', *Population Studies* 39, no. 2 (1985): 281, table 8. This article is cited in Berry and Foyster, 'Childless Men in Early Modern England', p. 162. They read the data to refer only to whether or not women conceived within the first five years after marriage. However, the data in table 8 clearly refer to women who did not give birth at a specific age *or any subsequent age*, including information about women who never gave birth after their marriage. In fact, Trussel and Wilson state on page 285 that '4.6 per cent of this cohort [women who married between the ages of twenty and twenty-four] *never* had a child'.
25. Gowing, *Gender Relations in Early Modern England*, p. 22.
26. C.S. Knighton, 'Pepys, Samuel (1633–1703)', in *Oxford Dictionary of National Biography, Online ed.*, ed. Lawrence Goldman (Oxford: Oxford University Press, 2004).
27. Edward Gregg, 'Anne (1665–1714),' in *Oxford Dictionary of National Biography, Online ed.*, ed. Lawrence Goldman (Oxford: Oxford University Press, 2004).
28. Eucharius Roesslin, *The Byrth of Mankynde Newly Translated out of Laten into Englysshe, Etc.* (London: Thomas Raynalde, 1540). Audrey Eccles, *Obstetrics and Gynaecology in Tudor and Stuart England* (Kent, OH: Kent State University Press, 1982), pp. 11–15.
29. Merry E. Wiesner, *Christianity and Sexuality in the Early Modern World: Regulating Desire, Reforming Practice* (London Routledge, 2010), pp. 43–46, 104–107. Ronnie Po-chia Hsia, *The World of Catholic Renewal, 1540–1770* (Cambridge: Cambridge University Press, 1998), pp. 41–42.

30. Ulinka Rublack, 'Pregnancy, Childbirth and the Female Body in Early Modern Germany', *Past & Present*, no. 150 (1996): 87. Anthony Fletcher, 'The Protestant Idea of Marriage in Early Modern England', in *Religion, Culture, and Society in Early Modern Britain: Essays in Honour of Patrick Collinson*, ed. Patrick Collinson, Anthony Fletcher and Peter Roberts (Cambridge Cambridge University Press, 1994). Crawford, *Blood, Bodies, and Families in Early Modern England*, p. 83.
31. Mary Fissell, 'The Politics of Reproduction in the English Reformation', *Representations* 87, no. 1 (2004): 43–81.
32. Walsham, *Providence in Early Modern England.*
33. Monica Helen Green, *Making Women's Medicine Masculine: The Rise of Male Authority in Pre-Modern Gynaecology* (Oxford: Oxford University Press, 2008). Helen King, *Midwifery, Obstetrics and the Rise of Gynaecology: The Uses of a Sixteenth-Century Compendium* (Aldershot: Ashgate, 2007).
34. Alexandra M Lord, '"The Great Arcana of the Deity:" Menstruation and Menstrual Disorders in Eighteenth-Century British Medical Thought', *Bulletin of the History of Medicine* 73, no. 1 (1999): 39–41.
35. Patricia Crawford, *Women and Religion in England 1500–1720* (New York: Routledge, 1993): pp. 82–83.
36. Gowing, *Gender Relations in Early Modern England*, p. 83.

CHAPTER 2

Experiencing Infertility

When Rowland Wilson died in 1650, his wife Mary was still young, and a widow of some means. She caught the attention of several suitors, among them Bulstrode Whitelocke. Mary described Bulstrode in her memoirs as 'a grave gentleman that had ten children, which at the first notion did startel me and did cause all my friends to be against it [the match]'.[1] After some consideration, however, Mary accepted Bulstrode's proposal, deciding that if children were a divine blessing, then she 'darst not refuse a man for having ten blessings, nay though he told me he would settel all his estate upon his other children'. Being childless for so long, Mary Whitelocke took some comfort in the possibility of becoming a stepmother, believing that 'in marrying him . . . [she] . . . might be in a cappassity to doe some good amongst those children'.[2] There was no practical reason for Mary and Bulstrode to have children together. Bulstrode had no need for additional heirs, and made it clear to Mary that should they have children together they would not inherit his estate. Mary also had no shortage of either the duties or the pleasures of motherhood, as she was charged with caring for Bulstrode's children, nine of whom were under the age of fifteen at the time of their marriage. Nonetheless, Mary continued to pray for a child of her own. She noted that she 'did beg of god very much in the time I was so long without any child that if ever he would give me a child that he would be a pleased to make it his child, and I did promis to god that if ever he should give me a child I would doe what lay

D. Oren-Magidor, *Infertility in Early Modern England*,
Early Modern History: Society and Culture,
DOI 10.1057/978-1-137-47668-5_2

in my power to bring him up in the fear of the Lord and to dedicate him to his servise'.[3] Regardless of any practical concerns, Mary Whitelocke wanted to become a mother in body as well as in name.

In one of the most significant studies of the history of the family in England, Alan Macfarlane states that couples in sixteenth- and seventeenth-century England desired children, but that they were wanted as 'an added pleasure' to life, amusing playthings that mirrored their parents and were nice to have around.[4] According to Macfarlane, there was little pressure on couples to bear children either in order to perpetuate a family name or for religious reasons, and certainly not in order to maintain their social standing.[5] It is true, as Macfarlane argues, that men and women were not judged on their ability to have as many children as possible, and indeed overly large families were frowned upon. It is also true that childlessness was not the biggest tragedy that could befall a woman in early modern England. Nonetheless, Macfarlane's analysis underestimates the social and religious significance of childbearing for married men and women in this period. It tends to trivialize the intense desire for children that many people felt, by stating that a main reason for having children was 'as playthings'. Whitelocke had as many amusing 'playthings' as she could want once she married Bulstrode, yet she still desired a child of her own. Other women and men expressed their desire for a child with a similar depth of emotion.

Macfarlane points out that there was no 'abuse or anger at childless women' in this period, suggesting that childlessness was not a disaster.[6] But this lack of abuse was not taken for granted, and women did have some expectation that their husbands would blame them, if not outright disdain them, for their childlessness. Whitelocke wrote of her first husband that he was so caring that he 'did never abraid me with the want of children', while Margaret Cavendish praised her husband for not wavering in his love for her, despite her infertility.[7] That Whitelocke and Cavendish felt the need to state this outright indicates that there was some existing idea that a husband was within his rights to be angry at a wife who did not bear him children. In short, infertility may have been merely a misfortune rather than a tragedy, as Macfarlane suggests, but as a misfortune it nonetheless had a profound impact on people's emotions.

Patricia Crawford argues that childbearing was particularly important for Nonconformist families after the Restoration in 1660, such as the family of Philip and Katherine Henry.[8] Forbidden to preach their beliefs outside the home, 'Puritan' preachers such as Philip Henry focused instead on their own families and households, aiming to make them bastions of good 'godly' conduct. In these families childbearing was crucial, because 'the births of children multiplied the number of Christians who would continue to witness to the tradition of their forbears'.[9] In such families, 'there was no greater misfortune than the barrenness of a wife'.[10] The Restoration may have had a particular impact on the significance of childbearing within families of this particular milieu, but this was actually only one instance of a broader world view that identified childbearing as women's avenue to salvation.[11] Childbearing was also meaningful as part of the social identity of both men and women, and within months of marriage friends and family members of the newly-weds might inquire as to whether the wife was pregnant.[12]

Childbearing was not a woman's only role in this society. Women managed households and estates, engaged in philanthropic work and provided medical care and nursing. They also laboured in fields, workshops and market stalls alongside men.[13] Women's work was sometimes similar or even identical to the work of their husbands, but the meaning attributed to this work was different. Men's work and activities were considered defining characteristics, even a vocation. Men were listed in tax records according to their profession, while women were listed by their familial connections—as daughters, wives, widows or spinsters.[14] True, many women did not marry, and more never became mothers, but the social and religious ideology gave women one central vocation: being a wife and a mother. This was both the ultimate expression of proper femininity and their avenue to religious salvation.[15] Therefore, while childless married women were by no means 'second-class citizens', they did fail to fulfil one of their central roles as women. Some childless women explicitly described their other activities in life as an alternative to bearing children. Many women engaged in 'good works', or helped to raise other people's children through fostering or informal adoption. The latter was part of the broad network of kinship ties which Naomi Tadmor describes, which functioned outside the nuclear family.[16] Indeed, fostering children or temporarily educating children of family members and acquaintances was quite common in early modern households.[17] Fostering could only be informal, because there was no option for legal adoption under English law until the twentieth century. Infertile couples could choose to educate and raise children, but they were unable to give them the benefit of legal status.[18] While many women engaged in such informal arrangements, as well as in philanthropic work related to education and other similar endeavours, childless women specifically described themselves, or were described by others, as fulfilling these roles *because* they had no children, or at least as an alternative to childbearing.

Personal Accounts of Infertility

Both men and women in this period had a stake in reproduction, and wrote of their desire for children. The foci of these desires, however, were somewhat different. Childless men primarily expressed concern about the perpetuity of their family name and the inheritance of their property. They might continue to want children until they felt that this goal was secure, and then begin to worry that any additional children might be beyond their means. Childless women, meanwhile, described their childlessness in emotional and religious terms. They saw motherhood as an important part of their lives that went beyond the practical considerations of providing heirs to a fortune, a title or a kingdom, keeping the family bloodline alive or having working hands to keep the farm or the business going.[19] For women, infertility had a deeper meaning, going to the core of their identity. If they were devout, this meaning was clear: their infertility was meant to test their faith and to teach them to accept their lot in life. Their response was to rely on prayer to give them hope that they might bear children, while keeping faith that if they did not have children, this was part of a providential plan.[20]

Like many women in 'godly' communities, the prominent Puritan poet Anne Bradstreet left an autobiographical text for her children, written with the intent of providing religious guidance and advice.[21] Bradstreet described the religious course that led her to immigrate to Massachusetts in 1630 and the various trials of faith she had undergone during her life, among them an early struggle with fertility problems. 'It pleased God to keep me a long time without a child,' she wrote, 'which was a great grief to me, and cost me many prayers and tears before I obtained one, and after him gave mee many more.'[22] Bradstreet's reliance on prayer to understand and deal with infertility was quite typical of women in her social circle in this period. Quite possibly this was also the case for women of other religious persuasions, but they were less likely to leave detailed religious diaries and memoirs, so that their beliefs are more difficult to trace. Certainly religious sermons and manuals, written by clergymen of differing religious persuasions, suggested that a woman's proper response to infertility was to emulate Hannah, one of the barren women of the Bible, who prayed earnestly for a son; her prayer was answered. Infertile women took this advice to heart and saw Hannah as a role model.[23] In their study of childless men in the early modern period, Elizabeth Foyster and Helen Berry argue that the providential world view that saw infertility as a direct result of divine intervention, was powerful in the sixteenth century, but had lost much of its power by the eighteenth century.[24] However, the evidence in women's personal accounts of infertility indicates that some women were treating infertility as a personal test of faith even at the end of the seventeenth century, which accords with Alexandra Walsham's claim that Providentialism was eroding towards the end of the seventeenth century, but lingered in some ways even into the eighteenth.[25]

While some women left explicit descriptions of their struggle with infertility and the meanings they gave to it, in other cases these can only be inferred from the existing record. Lady Margaret Hoby, childless throughout her three marriages, wrote an extensive spiritual diary, in which she never spoke of her infertility directly. Nonetheless, the modern editor of Hoby's diary, Joanna Moody, argues that at least two instances in Hoby's diary likely refer to her fertility problems. In 1600, Hoby recorded consulting Mr. Lister, her physician, about 'some of my greues [griefs]'. Moody argues that the matter was likely a medical rather than an emotional one, because Hoby reserved spiritual consultations for her cleric, and that the vagueness of the entry indicates that it was a delicate matter, because Hoby wrote about other medical complaints without subterfuge.[26] Medical treatment for ailments was common even among staunch Puritans and was in full accordance with providential views, which believed that God brought about illness through natural means, which could then also be cured through natural means.[27] The treatment of infertility was no different, and it is not surprising that Hoby might have consulted her physician on the matter. The entry from 7 October 1603, by contrast, is religious in nature. Hoby wrote that 'this day I fasted untill Eueninge, eatinge nor drinkinge any thinge, begging of the Lord that blissne [blessing] w[hi]ch yet I want: the Lord Heare me for his Christs sack, amen'.[28] Again there is no explicit reference to childlessness, but Moody suggests that this it is likely the cause of Hoby's ardent prayer in this instance, and evidence from other women's diaries bears this out, as they also use vague references to 'certain matters' that are fairly clearly a reference to fertility problems.

The most prominent example of such a diary is that of Sarah Savage, who lived almost a century after Hoby. Savage was Philip Henry's daughter and was raised within the Nonconformist milieu for which childbearing was of such significance according to Crawford.[29] Savage was married on 25 March 1687 to a widower with one daughter, and wrote about her wedding night a few days later. She expressed a hope that God would help her fulfil her new roles 'to discharge of duties as a wife, a mother & a daughter-in-law'.[30] For Savage, being a dutiful wife was connected with being a mother. On 22 May 1687, just two months after her wedding, Savage was already expressing a desire for children and a concern that perhaps she might not be fertile. 'This day a little desirous th[a]t God w[oul]d please to make me a fruitfull vine if hee see good,' she wrote, 'but if not I will submit to him.'[31] The metaphor of the 'fruitful vine' comes from Psalm 128:3: 'Thy wife shall be as a fruitful vine by the sides of thine house: thy children like olive plants round about thy table.'[32] Savage continued to be concerned with her fertility in later entries. In the entry for Friday, 10 June, she wrote 'That day and Satt[urday]. Had hopes th[a]t my God w[oul]d hear my prayer in a Particular matter yet still I referr the matter wholly to him,' while on the Sunday she noted having some impatient thoughts, because she feared disappointment.[33] It is likely that the 'particular matter' was that of childbearing, because when she was concerned with other matters, such as the health or spiritual well-being of a family member, Savage referred to them explicitly. Furthermore, as Crawford argues, Savage's recurring mention of a 'fear of disappointment' was timed in such a way that it was likely to coincide with her monthly cycle.[34] On 19 July Savage again wrote of disappointment: 'had hopes still t[ha]t God will grant the Lawf[ull?] desires of my soul as far as is good for me yet I trust all my concernments with him, desiring to bee ready for disappointments'.[35] In September Savage claimed to have reached a certain degree of acceptance about God's hand in the matter of her fertility. She wrote: 'I have attained to a good degree of satisfaction that if God sh[oul]d deny mee the mercy of children . . . it is in infin[ite] wised[om] if hee totally deny it it is in mercy & in love to my soul and hee see good to bestow it hee will. In the mene time, it is good for mee to hope & quietly to wait upon him.'[36] Perhaps it was a sentiment that Savage felt she ought to feel rather than one she found truly convincing, because she repeated it several times, including on 16 October, when she once again wrote of her willingness to wait for children and the submission to God's will should he choose to delay or deny her the blessing of offspring.[37] Savage's account demonstrates how quickly a woman might believe herself infertile after marriage, and how anxious she might be to have a child. Faced with the fear of infertility, Savage followed the advice given in religious guidebooks, by praying on the one hand and practising acceptance (albeit with difficulty) on the other. Despite initial disappointments in the form of an early miscarriage and the loss of a prematurely born son within days of his birth, Savage eventually gave birth to nine children, although only four would survive her.[38] Some of her worry about childbearing can be understood in the context of the familial pressures that Crawford describes. In the Henry family, childbearing was so much a central part of a woman's religious duty that even months within marriage the pressure to conceive was immense.

It is significant that both Hoby and Savage wrote about their childlessness in a veiled manner, while Whitelocke and Bradstreet wrote of it explicitly. Whitelocke and Bradstreet were writing after the fact, and were crafting narratives for their children to read. They could tell a clear tale in which they responded to infertility with prayer, faith and hope, and were rewarded by God with the children they desired. Hoby and Savage, on the other hand, were writing ongoing spiritual diaries. They did not know when and if their struggle to bear children would end, and might have feared to speak of it too directly, less they overstate their desires and appear to be demanding a child rather than hoping for one, something religious authors warned women to avoid.[39]

There is little evidence that couples abandoned hope that they would bear children, even after years of marriage. In some cases these hopes were justified. The Duchess of Lennox was treated for infertility for over ten years, seeking advice from the celebrated physician Théodore de Mayerne, before she finally became a mother.[40] The continued hope for a child did not just mean praying, or even seeking medical care. It also meant including the prospect of children in financial plans and life decisions. In his autobiography, statesman Sir William Trumbull noted that in 1684 he had to decide whether to take a position that would give him status and a sense of duty, but would also be a financial burden. At the time, he had been married for fourteen years with no children, and must surely have had some doubts as to his wife's fertility, if not his own. Nonetheless, Trumbull considered his new position in light of the financial burden that he might face should he become a father. He wrote of the various factors that influenced his decision, including his brother's debts, and the fact that his wife, Elizabeth, was 'Young, and tho it please god to give us no child at that time, yet it was probable enough that my family might be increased'.[41] After fourteen years of involuntary childlessness, Trumbull still considered it 'probable' that he and Elizabeth would have children. It was obvious to him that having children was a part of their married life. Elizabeth and William had no children during the thirty-four years of their marriage. William remarried after Elizabeth's death in 1704, and although he was already sixty-seven at the time, he had a girl and a boy with his second wife, Judith.

Childbearing was never only a 'women's issue', despite the deeper emotional investment that women expressed in childbearing.[42] One member of the Verney family, who had suffered a miscarriage during her first pregnancy, wrote when she had conceived again and was past the point when she was likely to miscarry again, that her husband was 'extreem fond of me since I was with child, he was ever a very kind husband to me, but much more so since I was with child'.[43] The case of diarist Samuel Pepys also suggests that men worried about the practical implications of childlessness.[44] Like Trumbull, Pepys continued to hope for children even years after his marriage, but he seemed less sanguine than Trumbull about the possibility that he would have them. An avid recorder of every aspect of his life, Pepys regularly recorded his wife Elizabeth's menstruation, partially because she tended to feel ill and keep to her room when menstruating, and partially because he was interested in her fertility.[45] In January 1660 he wrote that 'my wife, after the absence of her terms for seven weeks, gave me hopes of her being with child, but on the last day of the year she hath them again'.[46] Like Trumbull, Pepys also considered the possibility of children in conducting his family affairs, but unlike Trumbull, he was far from confident that he would have them. In January 1662 Pepys discussed a potential marriage match for his brother, Thomas, and indicated that he expected Thomas to be his heir, 'considering the possibility there is of my having no child'.[47] This did not mean that he gave up hope that he would become a father, only that he conducted his affairs under the assumption that he would not. On 6 November 1663 he wrote that 'my wife was mighty-earnest with me to persuade me that she should prove with child since last night, which, if it be, let it come, and welcome'.[48] The subject of childbearing then recurred several times in 1663 and 1664, including an episode in September 1664 in which Elizabeth believed herself to be pregnant but was not (a case in which Pepys himself noted that he 'neither believed nor desired' her to be pregnant, although the reason is unclear).[49] While Samuel worried about matters of inheritance and finances, he also worried about the more ephemeral matter of preserving his family name. In April 1664 he noted that Elizabeth had gone to the funeral of his cousin, and added that 'it is a sad consideration how the Pepys's decay, and nobody almost that I know in a present way of encreasing them'.[50] He was worried that his family line would die out if no one, including himself, managed to have children.

The Pepys's childlessness was of interest to members of their family, as one particularly bizarre incident suggests. In May 1664, Elizabeth told Samuel that she had met alone with Samuel's uncle Wight, who had lost all of his children. During the meeting, Wight brought up 'her want of children, and his also, and how he thought it would be best for him and her to have one between them'. The uncle was willing to pay her '£500 either in money or jewells beforehand' and to make the child his heir. When Elizabeth flatly refused, Wight tried to claim that it had all been 'in jest'.[51] Elizabeth had previously complained that Wight touched her inappropriately, and Pepys indeed wondered whether his entire relationship with Wight was based on 'only his lust for her', a disappointment for him if it was true, as Samuel hoped that Wight would name him as his heir.[52] Perhaps because of the delicate balance of power between the two men, Samuel resolved to say nothing of the incident to his uncle for the time being, but rather to save the information in order to use it at the appropriate moment.[53] It seems he never did so, and indeed maintained at least a cordial relationship with Wight for years afterwards. Wight's offer was certainly inappropriate and does not indicate any general practice. The fact that he made it at all highlights the fact that the Pepys's infertility was something that was well known and discussed and that it was at least suspected that the problem was Samuel's, a belief bolstered by the fact he never had children with any of his mistresses. Wight saw Elizabeth as a likely candidate for this offer, believing that in order to fulfil the desire to become a mother, she might be willing to stretch the bounds of decent and acceptable behaviour.

Although women worried about infertility independent of the considerations of inheritance or perpetuating the family that might concern their husbands, it was not self evident that they should do so. *Sociable Letters* (1664) is a series of fictional letters providing social commentary, written by Margaret Cavendish, Duchess of Newcastle and one of the unique intellectual minds of her time.[54] In one of those letters, Cavendish mocked two women, Lady D.S. and Lady E.K., who were both 'Melancholy . . . for Want of Children'. According to Cavendish, the

Lady D.S.'s sadness and concern were somewhat justified, 'by reason [that] her Husband is the Last of His Family unless he Have Children'. Lady E.K., on the other hand, had 'no Reason why she should be troubled for having no Children, for though it be the part of every Good Wife to desire Children to Keep alive the Memory of their Husband's Name and Family by Posterity, yet a Woman hath no such Reason to Desire Children for her Own Sake'.[55] In the letter, Cavendish criticized married women who 'desire Children, as Maids do Husbands, more for Honour than for Comfort or Happiness, thinking it a Disgrace to live Old Maids, and so likewise to be Barren'.[56]

Yet *Sociable Letters* seems to reflect an idealized version of Cavendish, or perhaps what she thought she ought to express.[57] Certainly this account does not accord with Cavendish's practice in life. The second wife of William Cavendish, who already had both sons and daughters, she was childless throughout her life, but sought treatment for her infertility and hoped to have children. Unlike Bulstrode Whitelocke, who was clearly concerned that he would be unable to care for any children beyond the ten he already had at the time of his third marriage, William Cavendish was still concerned about the security of his title and estates. It appears that William, rather than Margaret, was the chief instigator of the Newcastles' hope for children. Margaret wrote that 'he having but two Sons, purposed to marry me, a young Woman, that might prove fruitful to him, and encrease his Posterity by a Masculine Off-spring . . . but God (it seems) had ordered it otherwise, and frustrated his Designs, by making me barren, which yet did never lessen his Love and Affection for me'.[58] In a period with extensive childhood mortality, William may have felt that two sons were not enough, and so he played an active role in seeking fertility treatments for Margaret. Whatever indifference she implicitly claimed through the *Sociable Letters*, Margaret herself was not unaffected by her childlessness, and she wrote of her literary pursuits as a method of leaving something for posterity, having accepted that she would not bear children.[59]

The Uncertainty of Childbearing

The pressure to have children was significant, and it was intensified by the fundamental uncertainty of early modern childbearing. High infant mortality caused anxiety about the ultimate outcome of any pregnancy.[60] This anxiety was exacerbated by the difficulty of diagnosing pregnancy and of clearly identifying the causes of any fertility problems.[61] There was, of course, a coherent and logical medical system which defined the symptoms of pregnancy, but medical authorities themselves recognized that these were not absolute and that misdiagnoses could occur in both directions. Astrological physician Simon Forman stated that 'It is the difficultest thinge in Judgement to knowe whether a woma[n] be with child or not. For . . . a woman may have her courses and be with child and sometimes they have not their courses and yet are not with child. And sometimes again they are with child when they have not their courses.'[62] Lisa Smith argues that menstruation was not understood as merely reproductive in function, so that absence of menstruation was not immediately classified as either a sign of pregnancy or a fertility problem, but rather might be perceived as a general blockage requiring treatment.[63] As a result, women with a history of reproductive difficulties could not reliably know when they were pregnant, when their menstruation was irregular owing to medical problems or whether they were ever likely to bear healthy children. Because the reproductive body was seen as mysterious and difficult to diagnose, it was easier for couples to believe that they had fertility problems and to worry about their chances of bearing children if they did not conceive immediately after marriage. Women expressed their concerns about childbearing in their diaries and letters.[64]

Writing about pregnancy in this period, Cathy McClive notes that 'uncertainty was . . . a medical and physical reality experienced by early modern women and recorded by their medical practitioners'.[65] Diagnosis relied to a large extent on the patient's own description of her symptoms, in conjunction with various visual cues. These methods were problematic, and patients sought more definitive methods of diagnosing fertility and pregnancy. Midwifery manuals contained several examples of urine tests which were supposed to diagnose whether a person was fertile or not and whether a woman was pregnant, and there is evidence that such urine tests were also put into practice, primarily by unlicensed medical practitioners.[66] In most cases, however, pregnancy was diagnosed by identifying a combination of symptoms: stopped menses, larger breasts and various indications in the colour and shape of the face. These were all uncertain, because other conditions could cause similar symptoms.[67] The most definitive sign of pregnancy was the 'quickening', the noticeable sensation of foetal movement within the stomach. This was usually understood as the determinant of pregnancy for legal purposes, such as granting 'the benefit of the belly' to condemned criminals.[68] However, even quickening was considered uncertain, as it relied on reports by the patient herself, and might also be mistaken for other symptoms, most commonly 'colic' or 'wind'.[69]

Even women with significant experience of childbearing could mistake the symptoms of pregnancy and believe themselves to be pregnant when they were not. Honor Plantagenet, Viscountess Lisle, hoped to give birth to a male heir with her second husband, Arthur, an illegitimate son of Edward IV. The two were married in 1529. Lady Lisle already had seven children from her previous marriage, while Arthur had daughters but no son. The Lisles lived in Calais and managed their English estates and relationships through correspondence, most frequently with John Hussee, their London agent.[70] Lady Lisle did not face the fear that she was infertile and had every reason to believe that she could conceive again. Moreover, as a woman with a great deal of experience with childbearing, she could justifiably think that she was competent to determine whether she was pregnant, and in 1536 she believed this to be the case and announced it to her acquaintances. On 27 November 1536 Hussee wrote individually to both Lord and Lady Lisle to congratulate them on her ladyship being 'so well sped'.[71] Beginning in mid-December, similar good wishes arrived from the Lisles' various friends and acquaintances. In some cases these were accompanied by gifts, including a stomacher from cloth-of-gold to 'cover a young Lord Plantagenet' and two bottles of waters from Avignon to aid a healthy pregnancy.[72] All seemed to be progressing normally and letters continued to arrive, especially from Hussee, wishing Lady Lisle congratulations and expressing hopes and prayers for the birth of a son. In the spring of 1537 Hussee started signing his letters with an expression of hope to hear that Lady Lisle had delivered. In April he wrote that he was 'longing sore to hear that your ladyship had a son . . . '.[73] By June Lady Lisle must have believed herself close to the time of delivery and entered her lying-in, as Hussee wrote that he was 'very glad to hear that her ladyship hath taken her chamber'.[74] In mid-July Lady Lisle still hadn't delivered, but Hussee maintained his optimism and continued to write of his hopes that Lady Lisle would have not only a son, but twin boys![75] By late August Lady Lisle herself had come to the realisation that she was probably not pregnant at all, and this news must have reached her agent. Most of Hussee's letters to Lady Lisle were quite business-like and impersonal. His frequent expressions of joy at her pregnancy were no doubt genuine, but they were probably also formulaic and expected considering their relative social positions. On 23 August, however, Hussee wrote Lady Lisle a letter that broke entirely from his usual style and demonstrates the degree to which the false pregnancy had affected her and her acquaintances. Hussee attempted to maintain an optimistic tone, noting that Lady Lisle was not the first woman to have miscalculated the time of her conception. Nonetheless, he admitted that it was possible that all was not well, and advised Lady Lisle that she should not be too hurt if this was the case but rather put her faith in God:

> For if it be his pleasure he spareth neither Empress, Queen, Princess nor Duchess, but his handiwork must be suffered and his mercy abiden; and whatsoever is said or thought by any creature, God's works cannot withstand.[76]

It is hardly surprising that Lady Lisle was upset that her pregnancy turned out to be false. Hussee wrote that he had heard that her ladyship 'weepeth and sorroweth without comparison'.[77] It must have been particularly difficult when she had already received gifts, made preparations and even taken to the lying-in chamber to realize that she would not have a child. After this letter from Hussee, there are almost no explicit references to the pregnancy, and Lady Lisle never had children with her second husband. The fact that she was close to forty years old at the time of their marriage may have made childbearing both urgent and unlikely for her. The personal desire for children and the pressure of the intense interest from family and friends made it difficult to deal with the failure to have a child, even for a woman who was already a mother.

The difficulty in clearly identifying whether a woman was pregnant increased the sense of anxiety around reproduction and made it difficult to deal with fertility problems. This was particularly true for women who did conceive, sometimes frequently, but then suffered from miscarriages, stillbirths or premature labours resulting in the death of the infant. In those cases, women might see some of the symptoms of pregnancy, but would still worry about the viability of the pregnancy and the likelihood that it would end with a living, healthy baby. This was the case for Queen Anne, who was pregnant seventeen times during her life, but only had three children who lived past the first hours after the birth, all three of whom died during their childhood. Anne was not 'infertile' in any strict sense of the word, since she was able to conceive and had even carried several pregnancies to full term. However, her repeated miscarriages, stillbirths and premature labours resulting in the death of the child, together with menstrual irregularity, caused Anne to be constantly worried about her childbearing and uncertain about whether she was fertile and would be able to have more children. In July 1692 Anne wrote to her closest friend, Sarah Churchill, Duchess of Marlborough, to discuss the likelihood that she might be pregnant again after a previous miscarriage. 'I have not yet seen Lady Charlott,' she wrote, 'which I wonder very much at for I used to be very regular, & I cannot fancy she has taken her leave for nine months...'[78] Charlotte was neither a mutual friend nor one of Anne's ladies-in-waiting. Rather, she was a thinly veiled reference to Anne's menstruation, and Anne's anxiety about Charlotte signified her uncertainty about her own fertility. Charlotte's absence could signify a pregnancy, but it could also signify some reproductive disorder, or even the end of Anne's reproductive years. Anne and Churchill devoted a considerable portion of their correspondence to discussions of reproduction. They mentioned menstruation as a sign of fertility and the lack of menstruation as an ambiguous sign of either menopause or pregnancy. They discussed pregnancies, miscarriages and stillbirths. They worried about childbirth and they shared those worries with one another. A few days after this letter, Anne wrote again, and her concern about 'lady Charlott's' absence had grown, because the passage of time made her irregularity more pronounced. 'I am at this time in a very spleenatick way,' she wrote, 'for Lady Charlott is not yet com to me & I doubt if I should prove w[i]th child tis so soon after my illness to hope to go on with it... if I am not tis a very ugly thing to be so eregular...'[79] Anne relied on her previous experiences with pregnancy and miscarriage in order to understand whether her period was late because she was pregnant, because of a medical problem or because she was reaching the end of her fertile years. When she wrote that 'since my first three children I have never bred so soon', she was referring to the fact that she had only recently lost a child and did not believe it was likely for her to be pregnant again already.[80] Moreover, given her reproductive history, even a fairly certain identification of pregnancy could not give Anne a degree of assurance that she would have a living child.

Miscarriages and stillbirths evoked complex emotions in couples seeking to have a child. They were tragic disappointments, but they were also understood as a hopeful sign, evidence that the wife was able to conceive and that a future pregnancy might be more successful. It was a sign that 'though God hath taken away your little one to himselfe as the first fruites, yet I doubt not but he will hereafter blesse your wombe with children', as one seventeenth-century author wrote in order to console an acquaintance who had lost her child.[81] When Catherine of Braganza, wife of Charles II, miscarried in 1668, Charles wrote to his sister that he was 'troubled at it, yet I am glad that 'tis evident she was with child, which I will not deny to you till now I did fear she was not capable of'. He hoped that in a future pregnancy, Catherine's physicians would be able to treat her to prevent a recurrence of the difficulty.[82]

Miscarriage was particularly difficult for childless couples, for whom the stakes of reproduction were high. However, women who already had living children were also shaken by them, and sought to explain and understand them as part of a divine plan. The prayer book of Elizabeth, Countess of Mordaunt, contained a prayer of thanksgiving following a miscarriage in 1673. She thanked God for helping her survive through the miscarriage and its aftermath, and expressed gratitude for the reminder of 'the afflications and the mercis I have reseved from the Allmighty hand'. She saw the miscarriage as a reminder of her sins and a call to improve her ways.[83] In 1657, Mary Carey, the mother of seven healthy children, miscarried. The event moved her sufficiently to write a poem, entitled 'Upon the Sight of My Abortive Birth: The 31st of December 1657'. For Carey, the miscarriage was as much an act of divine goodness as the birth of her living children. She wrote:

> What birth is this: a poor despised creature?
> A little embryo, void of life and feature.
> Seven times I went my time . . . and mine all living . . .
> That was great wisdom, goodness, power, love,
> praise to my dear Lord . . .
> this is no less. The same God hath it done.

Through the miscarriage, Carey learned to submit her will to that of God, which is 'more dear to me than any Child'. Furthermore, she claimed that she found joy in the fact that God had another innocent soul with him in heaven.[84] As with infertility itself, miscarriages were understood within a divine plan, as reminders to submit to providence and accept God's will.

Even outside 'godly' rhetoric, miscarriages were used to criticize and censure women for improper conduct. If a woman miscarried, it was implied that she had done something wrong during her pregnancy, and that she must conduct herself more appropriately in the future.[85] After Elizabeth Cadogan, the daughter of famed physician Hans Sloane, miscarried in 1723 her physician suggested that this was due to excessive walking the day before.[86] Princess Mary (later Queen Mary II) was advised by her father, James II, to 'pray let her be more careful of herself another time' after a miscarriage in 1678.[87] And when Henrietta Maria, wife of Charles I, was pregnant again after a miscarriage in 1630, her mother sent her a chaise carriage to ensure that she travelled in safety. Henrietta Maria 'hope[d] God may grant me the favor to go to the end of my term', but promised that 'as to what depends upon me, I shall take all possible care of myself'.[88] Charles added a further note to Henrietta Maria's letter to her mother, thanking her for the gift, and assuring her that 'thank God, she is so careful of herself that I have no need to use other authority than that of love' to persuade Henrietta Maria to be careful.[89] There was an implication here that the women were themselves responsible for miscarriages by not placing the care of their pregnancy at the top of their priorities, and instead going out or being excessively active in ways that were perhaps improper for 'breeding women'.[90]

All women might be subjected to this form of criticism and policing, but royal women were, of course, much more susceptible to public and private scrutiny regarding their reproduction. The entire kingdom had a stake in their ability to bear children, and so the questions of whether the queen had conceived, how successful her pregnancy had been and whether she had given birth to a living child were of the utmost importance. No case proves this better than the Warming-Pan Scandal of 1688, involving James II and his second wife, Mary of Modena. Mary had suffered from recurring fertility problems during their marriage, before announcing in 1688 that she had given birth to a healthy male heir to the throne. This was a momentous announcement in political terms, because James and Mary were both Catholics and as James's children from his first marriage were both daughters, the son would become a Catholic heir to the kingdom and potentially restore Catholicism. The announcement of the birth of the Prince of Wales was a cause for concern for Protestants in England, and especially for the Tory-Anglicans who were already opposed to James's policies granting increased religious freedom while promoting the power of the king over that of parliament.[91] James's opponents began to circulate rumours that the pregnancy was fake or that the queen had miscarried very early on, and once the birth was announced they claimed that the living baby boy was not the royal heir, but a child that had been smuggled into the birthing room in a bed-warming pan, hence the name of the scandal.[92] The rumours that the pregnancy was faked were promoted and possibly even instigated by the princess Anne, who was dealing with her own reproductive problems at this time, and saw the birth of a male child as a threat to her own reproductive and dynastic hopes.[93] The matter of Mary of Modena's pregnancy was contested well after James II was deposed in the revolution of 1688. The younger James tried to claim the throne after his father's death in 1701, styling himself James III. Efforts to prove his illegitimacy therefore continued into the eighteenth century, with examinations made into the depositions of former witnesses on both sides of the debate. The examiners questioned Mary's former ladies-in-waiting, her apothecary and many of the people who had been associated with the court at the time, all with the aim of either proving or disproving her claims that she had carried a pregnancy to full term and given birth to a healthy prince.[94]

Following the scandal, the Bishop of Worcester, an enemy of the king, was questioned, and he attempted to use the spotty reproductive history of the royal couple as proof that the queen could not possibly have given birth to a son.[95] He claimed that 'in the years 74, 75, 76 she [Mary of Modena] had 3 children who all died within the compass of a year after their birth, the physicians concluded that there were *mala stamina vita* by reason of the dukes distemper, and that some being hereditary in her family in as high a degree or higher than in any family in Italy, and their could be no child to live. From 76 to 84 we heard of nothing but miscarriages.' In 1687 it was announced that the queen was with child, but 'the queen miscarried on Easter Monday' according to the bishop. His deposition intended to claim that it was impossible for Mary to have given birth to a viable son, as her reproductive history proved that she was inherently incapable of doing so.[96] Meanwhile Margaret Dawson, Mary's lady-in-waiting and one of those who consistently defended the birth of the Prince of Wales as real, noted that previously the queen had been unable to conceive, but that following her visit to Bath, there was an alteration in her temperament that allowed her to bring a pregnancy to full term. For Dawson, the queen's miscarriages were signs of a problem that needed to be fixed in order for successful childbearing to occur, and once this problem was managed, there was no reason to believe the pregnancy was false.[97] Dawson and the bishop both felt qualified and comfortable speaking about the queen's reproductive history, seeing it as a matter of general interest that was not limited to herself or her family.

Indeed, royal reproduction was a matter for general public commentary, outside courtly or political circles. In 1685 Hannah Stanhope, a member of the Yorkshire gentry, was visiting London. She wrote to her sister Mary that she had been several times at Whitehall to see King James II and his wife at dinner, and had also seen them at prayer. The queen, Stanhope noted, 'is a very handsome woman, but it is sertain she is not with child'. On the other hand, Stanhope reported that 'the prences Ann of Denmark was brought a bed this day of another daughter'.[98] Anne was the great reproductive hope for England's Protestants. Her elder sister, Mary, was believed infertile, but in 1685 it still seemed likely that Anne would bear a Protestant heir to the Stuart line. If Mary of Modena were not pregnant, while Anne was having children, this was of great importance to the public.[99] The pressures on royal women to bear children were huge, and their effect was personal as well as political. Pregnant for the tenth time, but with only one living child, Anne wrote to Churchill in 1693 that she was 'so desirous of children I would do any thing to go on [with the pregnancy]'.[100] Like women lower down the social scale, queens and princesses felt the desire for children as a personal hope, and failed childbearing was an emotional blow.

Interest from Family and Friends

Most couples were not members of the royal family, and their reproductive failures and successes were not subject to the same extensive scrutiny, but they were nonetheless of interest to the their kin and friends. Lisa Smith argues that in early modern France 'the infertility of any woman was of tremendous interest to her family, friends and neighbours' and that 'the public nature of reproduction was not unique to the high and mighty', because 'bodies, illness and reproduction all had social meanings beyond the individual'.[101] This was equally true in England, where within months of marriage a couple might be asked about signs of a pregnancy and friends and relatives would assume that childbearing was a priority for the newly-weds. In 1650, Jane Glanville gave birth to her first child. In a letter to her brother John Evelyn, she thanked him for his enthusiastic response to the news of the birth, noting that 'My happiness in being a mother is not a little increased by the joy you have therein.' She was also quick to wish the same joy upon her brother, who was married for three years and still had no children. 'When you have done itt [had children],' she wrote, 'you will quickly perseave that the mirrits of a good husband are att once . . . increased.'[102] Elizabeth Cope wrote to her sister Rachel Bourchier, Countess of Bath, in 1651 with news about her newborn son, William. At the time Elizabeth had three children, while Rachel had been married for many years but remained childless. Signing her letter, Elizabeth did not fail to wish Rachel 'a happy hour' of her own.[103] Men also expressed such interest in their friends' reproductive success. In 1697 Sir Hans Sloane received a letter from one of his acquaintances, naturalist John Ray. Ray noted that he had heard that Sloane's wife, Elizabeth, was ill. He expressed hope that the illness was the result of pregnancy, 'especially because I have not heard that you have as yet had any issue by her'. He added that he prayed she would make Sloane the parent of beautiful offspring, 'if she had not already done so'.[104] Sloane had been married in 1695, and the exact birth date of his first daughter, Elizabeth, is unclear, so he may not have yet been a father at this time. Regardless, it was obvious to Ray that within two years of marriage Sloane's wife ought to bear children, unless there was some problem.

This interest raised the pressure on childless couples and made their infertility more apparent, but friends and family could also provide support in a difficult time. Women's homosocial networks, in particular, exchanged medical advice and emotional support, while still remaining potent locations for gossip about reproduction.[105] One satirical piece against marriage entitled *The Ten Pleasures of Marriage* (1688) offers a fictional but interesting view of how such networks might have worked.[106] This work has sometimes been attributed to the prolific female dramatist Aphra Behn, but that attribution is now considered highly unlikely.[107] The work itself portrayed women's attitudes towards matrimony and fertility in an exaggerated and misogynistic way. Despite this, the satire does give a glimpse of the kind of concern that women, especially inexperienced women, could have about their ability to conceive and the success of their reproductive processes. It also suggested that such reproductive concerns were shared among women. *The Pleasures of Marriage* described acerbically the process by which immediately upon agreeing to marry, the wife wasted her husband's money and monopolized his time, instead of managing the household as she should. In the fourth chapter the couple finally planned to settle down after the courtship, wedding and a period of travel. However, the wife, rather than acting 'like a House-Wife' and beginning 'to order herself to take some care for the concerns of the Family', chose to go 'a prattling by her Neighbours; complaining of her barrenness, and takes Physick for it'.[108] The wife first began to display concern when she saw one of her neighbours playing with her child and the other preparing for childbirth. When a third neighbour, Mistress Maudlen, complained about her inability to conceive, the young wife realized that she has been married for three months without conception. At the encouragement of her neighbours, she began to believe herself or her husband infertile.[109] This 'Councel of women' then took it upon themselves to ask intimate questions about the young couple's sexual activities and married life in order to aid the bride with her complaints. The bride became so convinced of her fertility problems that anyone she speaks with 'pities her, and gives her their advice'.[110] Because this is a satirical piece against marriage, naturally the advice consisted of blaming the husband's sexual performance, and therefore he is the one who needed to be cured by consuming aphrodisiacs such as oysters, eggs and chocolate, but also by avoiding such 'drying things' as tobacco.[111] The husband himself tried to 'vindicate himself' using 'reasons and examples given by several learned Doctors; Culpeper; the Queens midwife; and some others'. Eventually, the husband was persuaded to 'take th'advice of [the] Doctor', while the wife was convinced to 'consult with some experienced Midwives and old Doctresses, to the end, that those distempers which are the occasion of barrenness, might be better removed and taken away'.[112]

While *The Ten Pleasures* is a fictional piece, there is some evidence that women did exchange this kind of reproductive gossip and advice. Cavendish's semi-fictionalized *Sociable Letters* contain several descriptions of women talking and gossiping about pregnancy and infertility, both their own and those of third parties in their social circle.[113] There is also such an interaction in Queen Anne's correspondence with Sarah Churchill, in which the two women shared information and advice about reproduction. On one occasion Anne, who was undergoing treatment to help her conceive and was yet unsure of its success, specifically asked Churchill not to share information about it with other women, especially the queen, Mary of Modena. This request suggested that women within a social circle would have discussed each other's reproductive problems. Some evidence of this social network of women exchanging reproductive advice appears in the margins of fertility recipes collected in women's private recipe books. These contained medical recipes that were exchanged by women, and often contained marginal notes about the origin of specific recipes.[114] These notes provide evidence of how reproductive information circulated within women's networks.

Johanna St John's recipe book contains approximately forty reproductive recipes, half of which contain some attribution, either to a physician or to an acquaintance. Two of these are particularly revealing of the social information that was attached to fertility-related recipes, and they list specific cases in which the recipe had been used. One recipe to prevent miscarriage ended with the suggestion to take it 'at any time when any fright or disorder happens to you'. In order to demonstrate the efficacy of the recipe, St John noted that 'this made Mrs. Sands goe through'. Presumably Mrs Sands had been at a known risk to miscarry, making the fact that she carried her pregnancy to full term evidence of the recipe's usefulness.[115] Another recipe in St John's collection begins 'To Cause Conception, Mrs Patricke Conceived Twice together with it & she advised it to one that had been nine years marryed on whom it had the same effect.'[116] Knowing that other women of her acquaintance had used the recipes successfully allowed St John to evaluate how effective they were in comparison to other remedies in her book for the same conditions. The information is also revealing of the relationships that women shared within the social network that circulated medical knowledge. The statement that Mrs Sands went through her pregnancy successfully with the former recipe would have been more meaningful as evidence of the recipe's efficacy if St John knew that Mrs Sands had been suffering from reproductive difficulties. Similarly, the claim that Mrs Patrick conceived after the use of a recipe would be more useful as proof of efficacy if Mrs Patrick was believed to have some sort of difficulty in conception. Otherwise her conception might seem perfectly natural. The fact that St John included this information with the recipes is evidence that women did not merely circulate medical recipes without context. They also shared with one another more intimate information about their reproductive problems and how they had overcome them.[117]

Alternatives to Childbearing

Men were concerned about childlessness. It affected their ability to pass down property and preserve their family name. They desired children and likely had an emotional response to infertility, although they were less likely to express it explicitly. But regardless of how men were affected by infertility, it was not as central to their identity and the fulfilment of their social and religious duties as it was for women. Early modern women played many roles within the household and outside it. They managed the household, supervised labourers, participated in agricultural activities and also engaged in works of charity, medical care and more. But as Kenneth Charlton argues, 'of all the status-accorded roles for women, those of housewife and mother were pre-eminent'.[118] It was an accepted belief that childbearing was important to a woman's salvation, as well as her fulfilment of expected social roles.[119] This did not mean that childless women suffered from outright discrimination, but it did mean that childless women often sought ways to give their infertility meaning, and they did so by presenting their childlessness as an opportunity to engage more deeply in good works, religious activities, education and even literary or scientific pursuits. These were all activities that occupied many women of the upper classes, but childless women described themselves, or were described by others, as taking on these activities in lieu of childbearing.

Authors of spiritual guides for women advised infertile women to see their childlessness as a mixed blessing, allowing them to spend their time performing charity and caring for spiritual matters, since they could not be fruitful in body. New England preacher Cotton Mather recommended that a barren woman should recognize that her infertility 'causes her to be more *Fruitful* in all the good Works of *Piety and Charity*; more *Fruitful* in her Endeavors otherwise to *Serve her Generation after the will of God*; more *Fruitful* in all those things whereby *The Heavenly Father may be Glorified*'.[120] A treatise attributed to the Anglican clergyman Richard Allestree but published in 1694, thirteen years after his death, presented a more radical version of this claim. Allestree admitted that children were a blessing and that to be 'a joyful Mother of Children' was a sign of great favour, but he also suggested that this was extremely rare. Children were indeed a blessing but 'there is scarce any other Blessing, season'd with so much Acrimony of Misery and Danger'. He advised infertile women to think of the sorrows of motherhood and 'tell me, whether thy bemoan'd Sterility enjoys not more ease, and less sorrow?'.[121] The sorrows of motherhood, according to Allestree, included having wicked or deformed children, not having enough food to feed the children you have and losing children to illness, and suggested that all of these trials were more difficult to bear than sterility. Rather than moaning that she had no children, Allestree suggested that a barren woman should give her full love and attention to God, stating 'If Elkanah therefore could say to his Barren Wife, Hannah ... Why weepest thou? And why is thy Heart heavy? Am not I better to thee than ten sons? How much more comfortably may'st thou hear the Father of Mercies say to thy Soul, Why is thy Heart heavy? Am not I better to thee than ten Thousand?'[122] Allestree therefore suggested that infertile women should give a prayer of thanksgiving that God had chosen to make them barren and had thus 'kept me from that great pain and peril of Child-Birth which many have undergone' and had also enabled them to do more to serve both their husbands and God.[123]

Allestree's treatise seems insensitive and uncaring, but the basic idea that Mather and Allestree promoted was meaningful to some devout women, who expressed similar views.[124] Little is known about the poet An Collins, except that she published a collection entitled *Divine Prayers and Meditacions* (1653). It is possibly that Collins existed only as a pseudonym, but one of her poems presents what appears to be a heartfelt and genuine expression of the feelings of an infertile woman. The poem uses the seasons as metaphors for fertility, in which spring is normally the season of growth and fertility. However, writes Collins:

> But in my Spring it was not so, but contrary,
> For no delightfull flowers grew to please the eye
> No hopefull bud, nor fruitfull bough,
> No moderate showers which causeth flowers to spring and grow.[125]

Now that her 'spring' was almost past, with no fruits to show for it, Collins found acceptance of her situation, and even joy in the fact that while her body bore no children, her mind was

> Apt to produce a fruit most rare
> That is not common with every woman
> That Fruitfull are.
> A love of goodnesse is the chiefest plant therin
> The second is (for to be briefe) Dislike to sin.[126]

The view that childless women could and should focus on faith and good works could offer comfort, but it was also the inverse of a view that saw infertility as a sign of sinfulness. Even while religious authors encouraged women to pray for children, they also created a link between infertility in body and infertility in spirit. Samuel Hieron's *Helpe Unto Devotion* was published in numerous editions between its first appearance in 1608 and at least until 1650. It became one of the most popular works of piety in seventeenth-century England.[127] From its second edition, the book contained a prayer for barren women, which included the claim that infertility was deserved, a proper punishment for spiritual faults:

> Humble me (I praie thee) under thy hand, and grant that I may truely and sincerely, and feelinglie, acknowledge, that though this be no little crosse, yet it is nothing to that which I have deserved. It is just, I confesse with thee, to punish my barrennesse in grace, and my fruitlessnesse in holy things, with this want of outwarde encrease.[128]

This message too may have had some resonance for devout women. The private prayer book of Elizabeth Trumbull (d. 1704), wife of William Trumbull, was written in about 1684. As noted, at this time the Trumbulls had already been married for fourteen years with no children. The book contains no explicit mentions of childlessness. Whether Elizabeth had already given up praying for a child, or had simply not recorded those prayers, they were not written down in this collection. However, Trumbull did pray that God would teach her love and faith, while at the same time asking 'how sayest thou that thou lovest me if I have noe more love unto thee & I be so barren and fruitless in good works'.[129] It is possible that Trumbull was merely using this language metaphorically, but it is an interesting choice from an infertile woman, and follows on the tone of Hieron's claims that a devout woman must acknowledge that her infertility might be a punishment for spiritual transgressions.

Elizabeth Trumbull remained very active in other fields of her life. She travelled with her husband on his diplomatic missions, first to France, where she took great interest in the preservation of persecuted Huguenots, and then to Constantinople.[130] She also took on the care and education of her nephew, John (Jack) Dormer, eldest son of her sister, Anne. Anne's husband Robert was abusive, and their son was generally described by his mother and others as taking after his father. Elizabeth and William nonetheless took Jack with them on their travels, in what might be seen as an act of charity and kindness both towards Jack and towards his mother.[131] While this was not mentioned explicitly in the correspondence between Elizabeth and Anne, caring for Jack was also an act of surrogate parenting which appears to have been a frequent choice for childless women in the upper classes. Katherine Hastings, childless throughout her forty-two years of marriage, was a deeply devout Protestant, who shared with her husband, the Earl of Huntingdon, a plan to create a model godly household. Several members of their family and social circle sent their children to be educated in this household. The first Earl of Essex entrusted the care of his three children to the Hastings on his deathbed in 1576, and they also cared for Thomas Sidney after his father's death a decade later, as well as several other youths.[132] The emotional ties between Hastings and the Sidneys were so close that diplomat and poet Daniel Rogers described Huntingdon as their 'second mother'.[133] Hastings prided herself in particular on her skills in raising young women.[134] One of the women she educated was Margaret Dakins, who later became Margaret Hoby. In her own godly household, Hoby took her cues from Hastings, and also took upon herself the care of several young women, essentially acting as a mother to them.[135] In addition to such informal adoptions, childless women might also choose to become stepmothers, marrying men with children who needed care.[136] It was fairly common for upper-class families in early modern England to send their children to other households for a time, and women who had children of their own also engaged in such activities, but a different meaning was ascribed to the actions of childless women who took an interest in education or raised young children. The inscription on a statue dedicated to Rachel Bourchier, Countess of Bath, whose sister was wishing her 'a happy hour' well into her marriage, hailed Bourchier for her political involvement, her religion, her 'genius exceeding that of a man' and yet also her 'motherly disposition'.[137] It then noted:

> And, tho she was childless, yet she was
> parent to more than a thousand Children
> whom in a very genteel manner she brought up,
> gave them portions, consecrated and even ennobled.[138]

Obviously meant to present Bourchier in the best possible light, the poem contrasted her childlessness in body with the work she did both in caring for several children of others and in donating extensively to Oxford colleges and other educational institutions. As with Mary Whitelocke, who wanted a child of her own despite becoming a stepmother to ten others, this 'surrogate mothering' may not have completely fulfilled these women's desire to have children, yet it seemed to be linked to it.

While interests in education or a focus on good works and charity might be the expected social choice for a childless woman of means seeking an alternate identity, there were other options. The most notable example is that of Margaret Cavendish, who used her status as a childless woman with grown stepchildren to 'excuse' her interest in the literary arts. In the letter to the reader at the opening of her *Poems and Fancies* (1653), Cavendish asked her readers not to censure her for her work, because 'first, I have no Children to imploy my Care and Attendance, and my Lords Estate being taken away, had nothing for Huswifery or thrifty Industry to imploy my selfe in'.[139] Unable to engage in the duties of a 'proper woman', then, Cavendish claimed she was free to engage in poetry. The connection between Cavendish's literary efforts and her childlessness was more than merely a facetious attempt to justify her 'idle' or 'unwomanly' pursuits. Instead, Cavendish saw her writing itself as an alternative to the children she could not otherwise have. A few pages later, Cavendish concluded an apologetic poem with these verses:

> An Excuse for so much writ upon my Verses
> Condemne me not for making such a coyle
> About my Book, alas, it is my childe.
> Just like a Bird when her Young are in Nest,
> Goes in, and out, and hops, and takes no Rest
> But when their young are fleg'd, their heads out peep
> Lord what a chirping does the Old one Keep.
> So I, for feare my Strenghlesse Childe should fall,
> Against a doore, or stoole, aloud I call,
> Bid have a care of such a dangerous place:
> Thus write I much, to hinder all disgrace.[140]

This description of her book as a fledgling leaving the nest is connected with Cavendish's view of her writing her physical legacy, which she leaves to the world in lieu of children. Knowing her body to be infertile, she expressed instead a concern that she would become 'barren in mind', losing the capacity to make her literary children.[141]

Conclusion

Margaret Cavendish professed her desire to live eternally in the memories of her friends and her readers, and used her literary works to do so.[142] Such pursuits were beyond the interests of most early modern women, for whom eternity, if it existed, was achieved in the physical realm through childbearing and in the spiritual realm through the salvation of their souls. Therefore, if they could have no children, they focused instead on the spiritual dimensions of prayer, charity and education. Faith was a central tool through which women understood and experienced their infertility. They sought medical aid and attempted to behave appropriately in order to prevent miscarriages, but ultimately they believed that their childbearing was in the hands of God. If they never had children, it was incumbent upon them to understand God's will in this choice, without questioning it. Reading women such as Sarah Savage expressing their complete acceptance of God's will in a matter so close to their hearts, it is difficult to take them at face value. This is particularly true for women who expressed joy and thanks at suffering a miscarriage, because it taught them humility. These descriptions can be seen as performative acts of faith from women who felt that this was the 'proper' response to their situation. Spiritual diary entries were modelled on samples in guidebooks, and so followed a particular format and expressed specific views.[143] The fact that devout childless women repeated their claims that they reached acceptance suggests that it may have been more difficult to face infertility with equanimity than religious manuals may have advised. Nonetheless, the significance of religion to women's experience of infertility cannot be underestimated. Early modern women understood childbearing as a religious duty, perhaps their most basic religious duty, and when they failed to perform it properly they understood this within the context of their faith. If they finally gave birth to a healthy child, this was God's will, the result of prayer and faith. If they never did so, they used religion to give meaning to their condition and to shape their view of it. Women from 'godly' circles were more likely to express these views explicitly in spiritual journals, but other women were exposed to similar providential beliefs and likely understood their infertility within a similar framework, even if they were less likely to write about it. Childless men were less likely to express their concerns about childlessness in personal or emotional terms. They were more likely to worry about the posterity of their family name or the inheritance of property and estates. If they were devout, and particularly if they were nonconformist, they might see childbearing as connected with ensuring the posterity of the 'correct' faith, and thus see childlessness as a failure to fulfil their religious duties.

Childless couples, both men and women, did not experience infertility in a void. Their reproduction was a matter of interest to friends and family members, who could offer support but also censure. Royal women faced particular pressures because it was incumbent on them to provide heirs to dynasties and kingdoms, but other women were not exempt from scrutiny. Women of all classes faced inquiries about whether they were pregnant. If they failed to conceive within a few months after marriage, they might become the butt of gossip. If they miscarried they might receive well-meaning advice, but also recriminations. It was assumed that they might have done something to cause their reproductive ailments, making reproduction a means of policing women and ensuring their proper conduct, in addition to an avenue for personal or emotional fulfilment.

Notes

1. Mary Whitelocke, *Advice for Her Son Samuel*, Princeton University RTC01 Ms. 226, unnumbered.
2. Whitelocke, *Advice for Her Son Samuel.*
3. Whitelocke, *Advice for Her Son Samuel.*
4. Alan Macfarlane, *Marriage and Love in England: Modes of Reproduction 1300–1840* (Oxford: Blackwell, 1986), pp. 56–57, 61.
5. Macfarlane, *Marriage and Love in England*, pp. 57–59.
6. Macfarlane, *Marriage and Love in England*, p. 61.
7. Whitelocke, *Advice for Her Son Samuel.* Karen L. Raber, '"Our Wits Joined as in Matrimony": Margaret Cavendish's *Playes* and the Drama of Authority', in *Margaret Cavendish*, ed. Sara Heller Mendelson (Farnham: Ashgate, 2009), p. 75.
8. Patricia Crawford, 'Katherine and Philip Henry and Their Children: A Case Study in Family Ideology', *Transactions of the Historical Society of Lancashire and Cheshire* 134 (1984): 39–73.
9. Crawford, 'Katherine and Philip Henry and Their Children',44.
10. Crawford, 'Katherine and Philip Henry and Their Children',45.
11. Patricia Crawford, *Blood, Bodies, and Families in Early Modern England* (Harlow, England: Pearson/Longman, 2004), pp. 79–112. Linda A. Pollock, 'Childbearing and Female Bonding in Early Modern England,' *Social History* 22, no. 3 (1997), 287–288. Olwen H. Hufton, *The Prospect before Her: A History of Women in Western Europe* (New York: Alfred Knopf, 1996), pp. 178–179. Merry E. Wiesner, Christianity and Sexuality in the Early Modern World: Regulating Desire, Reforming Practice, (London Routledge, 2010), pp. 63–64.

12. Crawford, *Blood, Bodies, and Families in Early Modern England*, p. 179. Pollock, 'Childbearing and Female Bonding in Early Modern England,' 287–88. Hufton, *The Prospect before Her*, pp. 177–78. Berry and Foyster, 'Childless Men in Early Modern England,' p. 179.
13. Merry E. Wiesner, *Women and Gender in Early Modern Europe* (Cambridge: Cambridge University Press, 2000), pp. 106–113, 117–119, 167–171.
14. Wiesner, *Women and Gender in Early Modern Europe*, pp. 103–104.
15. Wiesner, *Women and Gender in Early Modern Europe*, pp. 75, 78–79.
16. Naomi Tadmor, 'Early Modern English Kinship in the Long Run: Reflections on Continuity and Change', *Continuity and Change* 25, no. 1 (2010): 15–48. Leo Albert Huard, 'The Law of Adoption: Ancient and Modern', *Vanderbilt Law Review* 9 (1955).
17. Naomi Tadmor, *Family and Friends in Eighteenth-Century England: Household, Kinship and Patronage* (Cambridge: Cambridge University Press, 2001), p. 112.
18. CMA McCauliff, 'The First English Adoption Law and Its American Precursors', *Seton Hall Law Review* 16 (1986). Huard, 'The Law of Adoption: Ancient and Modern.'
19. Alan Macfarlane, *Marriage and Love in England*, pp. 51–58.
20. Daphna Oren-Magidor, 'From Anne to Hannah: Religious Views of Infertility in Post-Reformation England', *Journal of Women's History* 27, no. 3 (2015): 86–108.
21. For more on this genre see Jennifer Heller, *The Mother's Legacy in Early Modern England* (England: Ashgate, 2013).
22. Anne Bradstreet, *The Works of Anne Bradstreet in Prose and Verse* (Charleston, NC: A.E. Cutter, 1867), p. 5.
23. Oren-Magidor, 'From Anne to Hannah'.
24. Helen Berry and Elizabeth A. Foyster, 'Childless Men in Early Modern England', in *The Family in Early Modern England*, ed. Helen Berry and Elizabeth A. Foyster (Cambridge: Cambridge University Press, 2007), pp. 165–166.
25. Alexandra Walsham, *Providence in Early Modern England* (Oxford: Oxford University Press, 1999), pp. 333–334.
26. Margaret Hoby, *The Private Life of an Elizabethan Lady: The Diary of Lady Margaret Hoby, 1599–1605*, ed. Joanna Moody (Stroud: Sutton, 1998), p. 114.
27. Hannah Newton, *The Sick Child in Early Modern England, 1580–1720* (Oxford: Oxford University Press, 2012), pp. 96–97.
28. Hoby, *The Private Life of an Elizabethan Lady*, p. 194.
29. Harriet Blodgett, 'Savage, Sarah (1664–1752)', in *Oxford Dictionary of National Biography, Online ed.*, ed. Lawrence Goldman (Oxford: Oxford University Press, 2004). Crawford, 'Katherine and Philip Henry and Their Children', 41–42.

30. Sarah Savage, *Diary of Sarah Savage*, CCRO ZD BASTEN 8, 25 March 1687.
31. Savage, *Diary of Sarah Savage*, 22 May 1687.
32. Ps 128:3 KJV.
33. Savage, *Diary of Sarah Savage*, 10 June 1687.
34. Patricia Crawford, 'Attitudes to Pregnancy from a Woman's Spiritual Diary, 1687–8', *Local Population Studies* 21 (1978), 43–45.
35. Savage, *Diary of Sarah Savage*, 19 July 1687.
36. Savage, *Diary of Sarah Savage*, September 1687.
37. Savage, *Diary of Sarah Savage*, 16 October 1687.
38. Blodgett, 'Savage, Sarah (1664–1752).'
39. Oren-Magidor, 'From Anne to Hannah,' 92, 100.
40. Théodore de Mayerne, *Ephemerides*, BL Sloane MS 2074, f. 120v–21v.
41. William Trumbull, *Autobiography*, Library of All Souls College, Oxford MS 317, f. 19.
42. On male infertility see Berry and Foyster, 'Childless Men in Early Modern England'. Jennifer Evans, '"They Are Called Imperfect Men": Male Infertility and Sexual Health in Early Modern England', *Social History of Medicine* 29, no. 2 (2014): 311–332.
43. Miriam Slater, *Family Life in the Seventeenth Century: The Verneys of Claydon House* (London: Routledge, 1984), pp. 124–125.
44. Berry and Foyster, 'Childless Men in Early Modern England', p. 158.
45. Cathey McClive, 'Menstrual Knowledge and Medical Practice in Early Modern France, c. 1555–1761', in *Menstruation: A Cultural History*, ed. by Andrew Shail and Gillian Howie (Basingstoke: Palgrave Macmillan, 2005).
46. Samuel Pepys, *The Diary of Samuel Pepys,* vol. 3 (London: Harper Collins, 1995), p. 1.
47. Pepys, *The Diary of Samuel Pepys,* vol. 3, p. 12.
48. Samuel Pepys, *The Diary of Samuel Pepys,* vol. 4 (London: Harper Collins, 2000), p. 365.
49. Samuel Pepys, *The Diary of Samuel Pepys,* vol. 5 (HarperCollins, 2000), p. 277.
50. Pepys, *The Diary of Samuel Pepys,* vol. 5, p. 134.
51. Pepys, *The Diary of Samuel Pepys,* vol. 5, p. 145.
52. Pepys, *The Diary of Samuel Pepys,* vol. 5, p. 145.
53. Pepys, *The Diary of Samuel Pepys,* vol. 5, p. 152.
54. 'Cavendish, Margaret, Duchess of Newcastle upon Tyne (1623–1673)', James Fitzmaurice in *Oxford Dictionary of National Biography*, online ed., ed. David Cannadine (Oxford: Oxford University Press, 2004).
55. Margaret Cavendish, *CCXI Sociable Letters Written by the Thrice Noble, Illustrious, and Excellent Princess, the Lady Marchioness of Newcastle* (London: Printed by William Wilson, 1664), pp. 183–184.
56. Cavendish, *CCXI Sociable Letters*, pp. 183–184.

57. Sylvia Lorraine Bowerbank and Sara Heller Mendelson, *Paper Bodies: A Margaret Cavendish Reader* (Peterborough, Ontario: Broadview Press, 2000), p. 14.
58. Karen L. Raber, '"Our Wits Joined as in Matrimony": Margaret Cavendish's *Playes* and the Drama of Authority', in *Margaret Cavendish*, ed. Sara Heller Mendelson (Farnham: Ashgate, 2009), p. 75.
59. Sara Heller Mendelson, *Margaret Cavendish* (Farnham: Ashgate, 2009), p. xiv. Bowerbank and Mendelson, *Paper Bodies*, p. 14.
60. Linda A. Pollock, 'Embarking on a Rough Passage: The Experience of Pregnancy in Early-Modern Society', in *Women as Mothers in Pre-Industrial England: Essays in Memory of Dorothy Mclaren,* ed. Valerie A. Fildes and Dorothy McLaren (London: Routledge, 1990).
61. Andrew Wear, 'Medicine in Early Modern Europe 1500–1700', in *The Western Medical Tradition: 800 BC to AD 1800*, ed. Lawrence I. Conrad (Cambridge: Cambridge University Press, 1995), pp. 215–216.
62. Simon Forman, *Medical Treatise*, Bodl. Ashmole MSS 390, f. 190.
63. Lisa W. Smith, 'Imagining Women's Fertility before Technology', *Journal of Medical Humanities* 31, no. 1 (2010): 69–79.
64. Elizabeth Countess of Bridgewater, *Devotional Book*, BL Egerton MS 607. Arthur Searle, *Barrington Family Letters 1628–1632* (London: Royal Historical Society, 1983), p. 172. Pollock, 'Embarking on a Rough Passage: The Experience of Pregnancy in Early-Modern Society'.
65. Cathy McClive, 'The Hidden Truths of the Belly: The Uncertainties of Pregnancy in Early Modern Europe', *Social History of Medicine* 15, no. 2 (2002): 211, 209–227.
66. Jane Sharp, *The Midwives Book, or, the Whole Art of Midwifry Discovered* (London: Printed for Simon Miller, 1671), p. 163. Alessandro Massaria and Robert Turner, *De Morbis Foemineis, the Womans Counsellour: Or, the Feminine Physitian* (London: Printed for John Streater, 1657), pp. 119–120. Margaret Pelling, 'Thoroughly Resented? Older Women and the Medical Role in Early Modern London', in *Women, Science and Medicine, 1500–1700: Mothers and Sisters of the Royal Society*, ed. Lynette Hunter and Sarah Hutton (Stroud: Sutton, 1997), p. 72. Margaret Pelling, *Medical Conflicts in Early Modern London: Patronage, Physicians, and Irregular Practitioners 1550–1640* (Oxford: Oxford University Press, 2003), p. 210.
67. Sharp, *The Midwives Book*, p. 103. Jacques Guillemeau, *Child-Birth or, the Happy Deliuerie of Vvomen* (London: Printed by A. Hatfield, 1612), p. 4.
68. McClive, 'The Hidden Truths of the Belly: The Uncertainties of Pregnancy in Early Modern Europe', 212.
69. McClive, 'The Hidden Truths of the Belly: The Uncertainties of Pregnancy in Early Modern Europe', 214–218.

70. David Grummit, 'Plantagenet, Arthur, Viscount Lisle (B. Before 1472, D. 1542)', in *Oxford Dictionary of National Biography, Online ed.*, ed. Lawrence Goldman (Oxford: Oxford University Press, 2004).
71. *The Lisle Letters,* ed. Muriel St Clare Byrne, vol. 3 (Chicago: University of Chicago Press, 1981), pp. 525, 27.
72. *The Lisle Letters,* pp. 553–555, 71.
73. *The Lisle Letters*, ed. Muriel St Clare Byrne, vol. 4 (Chicago: University of Chicago Press, 1981), p. 138.
74. Lisle and Byrne, *The Lisle Letters*, vol. 4, p. 149.
75. Lisle and Byrne, *The Lisle Letters*, vol. 4, p. 153.
76. Lisle and Byrne, *The Lisle Letters*, vol. 4, p. 159.
77. Lisle and Byrne, *The Lisle Letters*, vol. 4, p. 159.
78. Princess Anne, *Letters to Sarah Churchill*, British Library Add. MSS 61414, f. 7. The letter is dated 28 July. The archivist has added the year 1692 with a question mark, so the year is not certain, although it seems plausible as Anne's pregnancy ended in April of that year.
79. Princess Anne, *Letters to Sarah Churchill*, British Library Add. MSS 61414, f. 11.
80. Princess Anne, *Letters to Sarah Churchill*, British Library Add. MSS 61414, f. 11.
81. Paggit, J., *Commonplace Book*, BL Harleian MS 1026, f. 34
82. Charles II, *The Letters, Speeches, and Declarations of Charles II* (Funk & Wagnalls, 1968), p. 219.
83. Elizabeth Viscountess Mordaunt, *The Priuate Diarie of Elizabeth, Viscountess Mordaunt* (Duncairn: Privately printed, 1856), p. 153.
84. *Flesh and Spirit: An Anthology of Seventeenth-Century Women's Writing*, ed. Rachel Adcock et al. (Manchester: Manchester University Press), p. 54.
85. Lisa Smith makes a similar claim regarding France in Lisa W. Smith, 'La Raillerie Des Femmes? Les Femmes, La Stérilité Et La Société En France a L'époque Moderne', in *Femmes En Fleurs, Femmes En Corps: Sang, Santé, Sexualités Du Moyen Age Aux Lumières*, ed. Cathy McClive and Nicole Pellegrin (Saint-Étienne: Publications de l'Université de Saint-Étienne, 2010), pp. 203–220.
86. *Letters to Hans Sloane*, BL Sloane MSS 4047, f. 19. Hans Sloane's correspondence has been extensively transcribed and documented in an online database: 'Sir Hans Sloane's Correspondence Online', https://drc.usask.ca/projects/sloaneletters/doku.php. This database was helpful in locating relevant letters.
87. W.A. Speck, 'Mary II (1662–1694)', in *Oxford Dictionary of National Biography, Online ed.*, ed. Lawrence Goldman (Oxford: Oxford University Press, 2004).

88. Mary Anne E. Green, *Letters of Queen Henrietta Maria, Including Her Private Correspondence with Charles I* (London: Richard Bentley, 1857), pp. 14–15.
89. Green, *Letters of Queen Henrietta Maria*, p. 15.
90. James Wolveridge, *Speculum Matricis Hybernicum, or, the Irish Midwives Handmaid* (London: Printed by E. Okes, 1670), pp. 106–107. *The Compleat Midvvife's Practice Enlarged* (London: Printed for Nathaniel Brooke 1659), p. 67. Gwynne Kennedy, *Just Anger: Representing Women's Anger in Early Modern England* (Bloomington: South Indiana University Press, 2000), p. 19. Gail Kern Paster, *The Body Embarrassed: Drama and the Disciplines of Shame in Early Modern England* (Ithaca, NY: Cornell University Press, 1993), p. 181.
91. For a more detailed discussion of the crisis and the revolution that followed it see Tim Harris, *Revolution: The Great Crisis of the British Monarchy, 1685–1720* (London: Allen Lane, 2006). Lois G. Schwoerer, *The Revolution of 1688–1689: Changing Perspectives* (Cambridge: Cambridge University Press, 1992). Steven Pincus, *1688: The First Modern Revolution* (New Haven, CT: Yale University Press, 2009).
92. M. Haile, *Queen Mary of Modena: Her Life and Letters* (New York: Dent, 1905), pp. 179–180.
93. Edward Gregg, 'Anne (1665–1714)', in *Oxford Dictionary of National Biography, Online ed.*, ed. Lawrence Goldman (Oxford: Oxford University Press, 2004).
94. On the political significance of the exploration of women's bodies in relation to the Warming-Pan Scandal see Rachel Weil, 'The Politics of Legitimacy: Women and the Warming-Pan Scandal', in *The Revolution of 1688–89: Changing Perspectives,* ed. Lois G. Schwoerer (Cambridge: Cambridge University Press, 1992).
95. *Depositions Pertaining to the 'Pretended' Prince of Wales,* BL Add. MSS 33286 f. 8.
96. *Depositions Pertaining to the 'Pretended' Prince of Wales*, f. 8.
97. Margaret Dawson, *Deposition on the Birth of the Prince of Wales*, BL Add. MSS 26657, f. 18.
98. Hannah Stanhope, *Letter to Her Sister, May 13 1685*, West Yorkshire Archive SpSt/6/1/17.
99. Gregg, 'Anne (1665–1714)'.
100. Princess Anne, *Letters to Sarah Churchill,* British Library Add. MSS 61415, f. 34.
101. Lisa Smith, 'La Raillerie Des Femmes?'.
102. Jane Glanville, *Letters to Her Brother John Evelyn, 1650–1651*, BL Add. MSS 78305, f. 27.

103. Elizabeth Cope, *Letter to Rachel Fane, Countess of Bath, September 12 1651*, KHLC u269/c273/6.
104. John Ray, *Letter to Hans Sloane, 1697*, BL Sloane MS 4036, f. 381.
105. Laura Gowing, 'Secret Births and Infanticide in Seventeenth-Century England', *Past & Present*, no. 156 (1997): 87–115. Pollock, 'Childbearing and Female Bonding in Early Modern England'. Sara Heller Mendelson and Patricia Crawford, *Women in Early Modern England: 1550–1720* (Oxford: Oxford University Press, 1998), p. 239. Adrian Wilson, *Ritual and Conflict: The Social Relations of Childbirth in Early Modern England* (England: Ashgate, 2016), pp. 155–156.
106. A. Marsh, *The Ten Pleasures of Marriage Relating All the Delights and Contentments That Are Mask'd Under the Bands of Matrimony* (London, 1682).
107. Mary Ann O'Donnell, *Aphra Behn: An Annotated Bibliography of Primary and Secondary Sources*, (Aldershot: Ashgate, 2004).
108. Marsh, *The Ten Pleasures of Marriage*, pp. 71, 73.
109. Marsh, *The Ten Pleasures of Marriage*, p. 76.
110. Marsh, *The Ten Pleasures of Marriage*, pp. 76–79.
111. Marsh, *The Ten Pleasures of Marriage*, p. 76.
112. Marsh, *The Ten Pleasures of Marriage*, p. 79.
113. Cavendish, *CCXI Sociable Letters*, pp. 94, 183.
114. Elaine Leong and Sara Pennell, 'Recipe Collections and the Currency of Medical Knowledge in the Early Modern "Medical Marketplace"', in *Medicine and the Market in England and Its Colonies, c.1450–c.1850*, ed. Mark S.R. Jenner and Patrick Wallis (Basingstoke: Palgrave Macmillan, 2007).
115. Johanna St. John, *Medical Recipes*, WL MS 4338, f. 213v.
116. Johanna St. John, *Medical Recipes*, f. 213v.
117. Daphna Oren-Magidor, 'Literate Laywomen, Male Medical Practitioners and the Treatment of Fertility Problems in Early Modern England,' *Social History of Medicine* 29, no. 2 (2016), 290–310. Leong and Pennell, 'Recipe Collections and the Currency of Medical Knowledge in the Early Modern "Medical Marketplace".'
118. Kenneth Charlton, *Women, Religion and Education in Early Modern England* (London: Routledge, 2002), pp. 33–34.
119. Charlton, *Women, Religion and Education in Early Modern England*, 124. Crawford, *Blood, Bodies, and Families in Early Modern England*, pp. 79–112. Pollock, 'Childbearing and Female Bonding in Early Modern England', 287–288. Hufton, *The Prospect Before Her*, pp. 178–179. Wiesner, *Christianity and Sexuality in the Early Modern World: Regulating Desire, Reforming Practice*, (London: Routledge, 2010), pp. 63–64.
120. Cotton Mather, *Ornaments for the Daughters of Zion, or, the Character and Happiness of a Vertuous Woman* (Cambridge, MA: Printed by S.G. and B.G. for Samuel Phillips, 1692), pp. 88–89.

121. Richard Allestree, *The Art of Patience and Balm of Gilead under All Afflictions an Appendix to the Art of Contentment* (London: Printed by R. Smith for E. Mory, 1694), pp. 111–112.
122. Allestree, *The Art of Patience and Balm of Gilead*, pp. 112–115.
123. Allestree, *The Art of Patience and Balm of Gilead*, p. 116.
124. *Flesh and Spirit: An Anthology of Seventeenth-Century Women's Writing*, pp. 16–17.
125. *Flesh and Spirit*, pp. 16–17.
126. *Flesh and Spirit*, pp. 16–17.
127. Vivienne Larminie, 'Hieron, Samuel (Bap. 1572, D. 1617)', in *Oxford Dictionary of National Biography, Online ed.*, ed. Lawrence Goldman (Oxford: Oxford University Press, 2004).
128. Samuel Hieron, *A Helpe Vnto Deuotion* (London: Printed by H. Lownes for Samuell Macham, 1611), p. 157.
129. Elizabeth Trumbull, *Prayer Book*, University of Birmingham Library 555, unnumbered.
130. Trumbull, *Prayer Book.*
131. Sara Heller Mendelson and Mary O'Connor, '"Thy Passionately Loving Sister and Faithfull Friend": Anne Dormer's Letters to Her Sister Lady Trumbull', in *Sibling Relations and Gender in the Early Modern World: Sisters, Brothers and Others*, ed. Naomi J. Miller and Naomi Yavneh (Aldershot: Ashgate, 2006), pp. 209–210.
132. Claire Cross, 'Hastings, Katherine, Countess of Huntingdon (c.1538–1620)', in *Oxford Dictionary of National Biography, Online ed.*, ed. Lawrence Goldman (Oxford: Oxford University Press, 2004). Margaret P. Hannay, Michael G. Brennan and Mary Ellen Lamb, *The Ashgate Research Companion to the Sidneys, 1500–1700: Volume 1: Lives* (Aldershot: Ashgate, 2015), p. 57.
133. Margaret P. Hannay, 'Mary Sidney's Other Brothers', in *Sibling Relations and Gender in the Early Modern World: Sisters, Brothers and Others*, ed. Naomi J. Miller and Naomi Yavneh (Aldershot: Ashgate, 2006), p. 97. Jan Van Dorsten, *Poets, Patrons and Professors: Sir Philip Sidney, Daniel Rogers and the Leiden Humanists.* (Oxford: Oxford University Press, 1962), p. 62.
134. Julie Crawford, *Mediatrix: Women, Politics, and Literary Production in Early Modern England* (Oxford: Oxford University Press, 2014), p. 86.
135. Hoby, *The Private Life of an Elizabethan Lady*, p. xviii.
136. Charlton, *Women, Religion and Education in Early Modern England*, 142.
137. Todd Gray, *Devon Household Accounts, 1627–59: Henry, Fifth Earl of Bath, and Rachel, Countess of Bath, of Tawstock and London, 1637–1655* (Devon and Cornwall Record Society, 1996), p. xxii.
138. Gray, *Devon Household Accounts, 1627–59: Henry, Fifth Earl of Bath, and Rachel, Countess of Bath, of Tawstock and London, 1637–1655*, p. xxii.

139. Margaret Cavendish, *Poems, and Fancies Written by the Right Honourable, the Lady Margaret Newcastle* (London: Printed by T.R. for J. Martin, and J. Allestrye, 1653), p. A7.
140. Cavendish, *Poems, and Fancies*, p. A8 v.
141. Bowerbank and Mendelson, *Paper Bodies*, pp. 14, 57.
142. Bowerbank and Mendelson, *Paper Bodies*, p. 71.
143. Avra Kouffman, 'Maternity and Child Loss in Stuart Women's Diaries', in *Performing Maternity in Early Modern England*, ed. Kathryn M. Moncrief and Kathryn Read McPherson (Aldershot: Ashgate, 2007), p. 172.

CHAPTER 3

Explaining Infertility

> In woman there maye be foure generall causes, by the whiche the conception may be impedyte and let [prevented]: over much callidite or heate of the matrice, over much coldnesse, over much humiditie or moystenesse, & overmuch drynesse. Any of these four qualities exceadynge temperancye, may be sufficient causes to lette due conception.[1]

This quote from the first midwifery manual to be printed in English, *The Byrth of Mankind* (1540), summarizes the causes of infertility within the context of humoral theory, the dominant medical theory of the premodern period. At face value, this quote indicates that infertility was understood purely as a physical ailment, caused by a distemper of the womb. If the womb was too hot, cold, moist or dry, then conception would not occur.

Most medical writing about infertility started with this basic model and expanded on it, but medicine was not the only explanatory model for fertility problems in this period. Another model guided Mary Whitelocke when she sought to explain her own history of infertility, one steeped in faith and providential theology. In her memoirs she described her first marriage as extremely happy and comfortable, noting that her husband was handsome, godly, kind and wealthy, and that 'our lives together was very comfortable and we wanted nothing that this word could afford'.[2] They were so content in their marriage that 'had not the lorde in wisdom

D. Oren-Magidor, *Infertility in Early Modern England*,
Early Modern History: Society and Culture,
DOI 10.1057/978-1-137-47668-5_3

and loving kindness for raisons best known unto himselfe withheld from us children w[hi]ch is the fruit of mariage: I think our lives would a been too happy'. Well versed in the providential theology of her time, Whitelocke saw her childlessness as a direct intervention from God. She believed that God had cast a pall on her worldly life by making her childless, so that she would lose her love for 'creature comforts' and instead focus on the spiritual life.[3] As Alexandra Walsham demonstrates, the belief in divine providence was mainstream in early modern English religion. Those who belonged to the 'godly' were more ardent in this belief, but the majority of English Protestants, regardless of their particular denomination, believed that 'God was no idle, inactive spectator upon the mechanical workings of the created world, but an assiduous, energetic deity who constantly intervened in human affairs.'[4] In this view, hardship was the method by which 'the Lord purged and proved His own', and God exercised His will in a veiled way, 'for the benefit and edification of human beings, to encourage due and grateful recognition of His wise provision for every contingency'.[5] Within this providential world view, infertility was to be understood as Whitelocke understood it, as a hardship which God in his wisdom inflicted upon the faithful in order to teach them humility, prepare them for salvation or correct their sinful behaviour and encourage them to repent. Devout men and women in this period understood their fertility problems first and foremost as acts of providence. God blessed unions with children, God took those children away if they died young, and if a couple had no children this too was according to God's plan. Some religious authors portrayed infertility quite vaguely as a trial or a cross to bear, without stating outright that it was a sign of misbehaviour. However, in other cases fecundity was explicitly described as a blessing and a sign of God's favour, while infertility was described as a punishment for sins. A treatise from 1591 described barren women as deprived of God's promise, and a sermon by John Hacket from 1675 stated that 'barrenness was a curse, and fruifullness of children a blessing'.[6] In a sermon on the occasion of the death of Emperor Ferdinand in 1564, clergyman Edmund Grindal highlighted Ferdinand's fruitfulness as a sign of God's blessing for his chastity. He contrasted Ferdinand with other princes, who 'living heretofore incontinently, have bene plaged of God with sterilitie and want of roial issue of their bodies'.[7] Donald Lupton argued that God threatened to give '*dry* breasts and *barren* wombs as a curse to *sinfull*, and *disobedient* Husbands', making women's bodies the terrain on which men were punished, to paraphrase Adrienne Rich.[8]

The two explanatory models, the religious and the medical, existed side by side. In itself this duality is unsurprising, and it can be explained easily by stating that the two models served different purposes, one to offer physiological advice, the other spiritual guidance, without directly competing one with the other. In such a view, the religious explanations for infertility might be seen as making a moral judgement, while medical explanations were 'morally neutral' about sterility, as Lisa Smith argues. Smith suggests that the medical view itself did not make moral judgements about infertility, but that medical knowledge could be used by laypeople in order to judge others.[9] Separating religion and medicine in this way, however, is a mischaracterization of the nature of early modern reproductive medicine. A close reading of medical guidebooks about fertility and pregnancy suggests instead that medical explanations of infertility contained within them an implicit moral judgement of infertile people, often by associating infertility with sinful conduct. Early modern medicine went far beyond the bounds of the purely physiological. A fundamental tenet of humoral theory was that a healthy body was one that was in balance, and that this balance was maintained first and foremost by moderation of the six non-naturals: air, food and drink, exercise and rest, sleep and wakefulness, excretion and retention, and the emotions.[10] When it came to reproductive health, moderation in sexual activity was also of crucial importance.[11] These were behavioural factors that patients could influence, but many of them also had moral, religious and gendered dimensions. When medical texts discussed the causes of infertility, they attributed it to modes of conduct which were perceived as immoral. Fertile couples were those whose bodies were moderately temperate and whose behaviour was controlled and commensurate with religious and cultural expectations of appropriate conduct. By contrast, patients who displayed morally reprehensible characteristics such as excessive lust, greed, gluttony and idleness risked infertility. It is not a coincidence that these were all 'mortal sins', a category that still held considerable sway even in Protestant England.[12]

Moderation itself, in all aspects of life, was the guiding principle of early modern moral ideology. The ideal of moderation drew from Classical origins, reinforced by the humanist rediscovery of Classical texts. It was a central tenant of moral ideology in both Protestant and Catholic countries and was incorporated into both religious systems, finding its way into English culture generally and into the Calvinist theology that founded important strains of English Protestantism specifically.[13] Moderation was also the defining characteristic of early modern ideals of masculinity. Men were expected to have self-control in all aspects of life, including sexuality.[14] In his study of moderation in the early modern English state and Church, Ethan Shagan offers an important reminder that moderation as an ethical system was not based on accommodation and toleration. Rather, it was based on aggressive social control and self-control. Moderation was not a passive avoidance of extremes, but rather 'the active force by which excesses were controlled and reduced to a mean'. In this period 'the ethical government of the self was understood as a microcosm ... of the political government of subjects'.[15] Therefore, when medical writers in early modern England highlighted the importance of humoral balance for health and fertility, and stressed moderation in sex, food, drink and emotions as the route to this balance, they were advocating a moral system that linked control over one's own conduct and emotions with conformity to a broader ethical, religious and social code of conduct. Indeed, Smith argues elsewhere that male infertility was expressly linked to venereal disease and debauchery in French medical texts, and that therefore 'male sterility ultimately emphasized a man's lack of self-control—something that men were ideally expected to possess'.[16] Medical explanations of infertility also embodied the gendered order, as Laura Gowing points out: 'A balanced body was the foundation of self-control, and self-control made it possible for men to live up to the commanding position required of them ... while the ultimate aspiration for the men who read bodily advice was to command others, that for women was to be able to be commanded.'[17] Reproductive advice promoted these ideas by highlighting the importance of properly controlled behaviour for both men and women in order to ensure fertility.

Medical authors were 'morally neutral' only in the sense that they rarely stated outright that infertility was caused by sinful behaviour or that infertile people were immoral. Their texts were firmly rooted in the internal logic of the humoral medical tradition, which was a coherent medical system in which certain behaviours and actions contributed to the imbalance of the humours and led to illness. Yet the behavioural factors that medical authors attributed to infertility were forms of conduct that were specifically censured by religious authorities and were connected with ideas of sin. Susanne Scholz argues that early modern behaviour manuals and conduct books gave advice on clothing, posture and carriage in order to 'inscribe a catalogue of virtues such as those provided by the writings of St. Paul and Augustine ... on the surface of the body'.[18] By associating infertility with cultural codes of conduct, medical guidebooks took this project of writing moral ideology onto the body a step further. How people *should* behave according to social and religious norms became how people *must* behave if they wanted to reproduce. Mary Fissell argues that midwifery manuals and childbearing guides were related to conduct books and other forms of prescriptive literature in the ways that they 'inscribe power relationships on the body'.[19] She suggests that such manuals worked to reinforce gender roles by positioning men as the active agents of the reproductive process and women as passive participants in it, and they may have done so, but they also went further. Midwifery manuals inscribed not only power relations but actual behaviours on the body, by linking the central goal of marriage—having children—with the appropriate behaviour of the married couple. The 'medical' explanatory model for infertility was therefore inextricably connected with the religious model, connecting moral and religious ideals to the very bodies of couples seeking to have children. Medical literature on infertility invited people to reflect on how their own behaviour influenced their ability to perform what was a central social and religious function: procreation. Just as medical texts drew from religious ideas and reinforced them, so religious ideology did not discount the role of medicine in understanding and healing infertility. Instead, the providential world view saw medicine as God's own creation, a gift to mankind, that could and would help to cure ailments, as long as this was according to God's plan.[20] The two models thus worked side by side to create the early modern understanding of fertility problems.

Humoral Theory

Humoral theory was at the heart of mainstream European medicine from ancient Greece and into the eighteenth century. According to this theory the body is comprised of four humours: blood, black bile, yellow bile and phlegm. Each of these humours corresponds to a set of two qualities: it is either hot or cold and either moist or dry. Each individual body has a proper balance of humours, with men tending to be hotter and drier and women tending to be colder and moister. Within this framework, illness is caused by an imbalance of the humours, and is cured by restoring that balance.[21] Within the humoral model, successful childbearing depends on both members of the couple having a proper balance of humours in their bodies and on the compatibility of their two temperaments to each other.[22] Therefore, the fundamental humoral explanation of infertility is the one that is quoted above, from *The Byrth of Mankind*: the infertile womb is either too hot, too cold, too moist or too dry. This explanation was taken directly from the corpus attributed to Hippocrates, and was then further elucidated and expanded by later authors.[23] Early modern midwifery manuals and guides to conception added additional information by looking at other causes of infertility beyond an intemperance of the womb, including the possibility of male infertility. They also went beyond explaining infertility to suggest methods of curing it. Learned physicians discussed reproductive knowledge in treatises written in Latin and intended for their own use.[24] This knowledge reached a much wider audience through the publication of popular midwifery manuals in English, which began in 1540 and expanded throughout the seventeenth century.[25] The content of these manuals varied, but the larger portion of each book was dedicated to descriptions of the reproductive system, advice for pregnant women and obstetric technicalities to be used during labour and delivery. Some books also contained a portion on the treatment of newborns, the choice of a wet-nurse and other post-natal considerations. All of the books also dedicated at least some small section to the process of conception and to potential reproductive difficulties, including inability to conceive, miscarriages and false pregnancies (known as 'molas').[26]

English translations of manuals in manuscript had appeared in the Middle Ages, including translations of the classic medieval gynaecological manual known as the Trotula, but their circulation was limited.[27] Printed midwifery manuals first appeared in the mid-sixteenth century, and the subject matter was quite popular. *The Byrth of Mankind* was a translation of a German midwifery manual which appeared when commercial English printing was still in its infancy. According to a survey of early modern English imprints, only ninety-two works were printed in English in 1540, of which thirteen were on topics described as 'medical, scientific, and utilitarian,' compared with 577 and thirty respectively in 1640.[28] Given the small number of imprints made that year, the decision to publish a midwifery manual suggests that this was expected to be a topic of some interest, likely to sell well. The book must have been successful, as Thomas Raynalde created a new edition of the translation and republished the book in 1545.[29] Throughout the late sixteenth century, and especially during the seventeenth century, numerous new titles were published in English, further indicating the reading public's interest in owning works that explained the basics of reproduction and fertility. Many of these books were adaptations into English from the works of Continental physicians, including Alessandro Massaria's *De Morbis Foeminis or the Woman's Counselour* (English edition in 1657) and François Mauriceau's *The Diseases of Women with Child* (translated and edited in 1683 by Hugh Chamberlain of the famous family of male midwives).[30] Others were original works in English, such as Nicholas Culpeper's *Directory for Midwives* (1651) or Jane Sharp's *Midwives Book* (1671).[31] Finally, there were also some anonymous compilations, such as *The Compleat Midwife Enlarged* (1656), which borrowed heavily from other published works both in English and in translation.[32] The popularity of midwifery manuals is evident not only in the range of titles, but also in the fact that many of them went through numerous editions and revisions. Culpeper's *Directory* had approximately ten editions in the first fifty years after its original publication.[33] The anonymous *Aristotle's Masterpiece* (1684), probably the most influential manual of the early modern period, went through at least twenty editions in the century after its publication and continued to be reprinted in dozens of editions throughout the eighteenth and nineteenth centuries.[34] Given their circulation and popularity, midwifery manuals played an important role in disseminating reproductive knowledge, at least to the literate portions of society, and they are therefore the most extensive source on how literate people understood fertility problems. While it is harder to identify what illiterate beliefs about fertility were, there is evidence that the medical knowledge within manuals circulated in some ways among those who could not read them directly. First, written works could be read aloud for more public consumption.[35] More significantly, medical knowledge could circulate through the work of informal medical practitioners, who might read some manuals and then promote some version of the knowledge within them in their own practices. This was certainly a cause for concern for physicians hoping to maintain their monopoly on medical treatment.[36]

The titles of midwifery manuals often identified the audience that they purported to address. Some, such as Culpeper and Sharp, addressed an audience of midwives.[37] Others wrote for a general female audience, or a mixed audience of laywomen and midwives, with titles such as *The Woman's Friend* (1666) or *A Companion for Midwives, Child-Bearing Women and Nurses* (1699).[38] In the front matter, authors expressed an intention to educate midwives in their profession and to teach women the fundamentals of conception, pregnancy and childbirth. Nicholas Culpeper explained that his *Directory* was intended to give midwives knowledge that the members of the College of Physicians were hiding from them.[39] Nicholas Sudell dedicated his *Women's Friend* to the ladies of London, claiming an intent to give women knowledge so that they could 'apprehend and perceive 1. What you are 2. What liable unto and 3. What assistance you have'.[40] While midwifery manuals were intended for a female audience, it is more difficult to ascertain who actually bought them and for what purpose. Certainly some women bought and owned them. They wrote their names on the books to indicate ownership and copied down recipes into their own private collections.[41] Midwifery manuals also appealed to some male readers, both because of their interests as husbands and potential fathers, and for purposes of titillation.[42]

It seems likely that infertile couples used such manuals to make sense of their condition, but the evidence of such usage is indirect at best. In the satirical work *The Ten Pleasures of Marriage* (1682) examined in Chapter 2, once the wife began to suspect that there was a medical problem, the husband tried to prove he was not at fault using 'examples given by several learned doctors; Culpeper; The Queen's Midwife [Louise Bourgeois, midwife to the queen of France, who was presented as a contributor to some of the anonymous compilations of gynaecological advice]'.[43] As a work of fiction, and more so as a satirical piece and one which drew on Continental sources, this is not direct evidence of actual practice, but its humour relied on the audience being familiar with the idea of using midwifery manuals to understand reproduction, and even with specific titles. Bridget MacArthur analyses both the origins of this text and its place within a genre of English satirical realism, that according to MacArthur, presents a fairly accurate and down-to-earth view of the attitudes of its time.[44] Stripping away some away the comedic and misogynistic elements, *The Ten Pleasures* does offer some indication of what couples with fertility problems would have done to deal with their condition, and this included seeking advice from popular midwifery manuals. This first and foremost explained the potential causes of fertility problems, while offering only some practical advice for curing them.

A couple looking at midwifery manuals in order to understand why they did not have children would have first learned about how conception worked and what hindered it. According to manuals, conception occurred when a man's seed entered a woman's womb and either combined with her seed (according to the Hippocratic two-seed theory) or was simply 'planted' in the soil of the womb to be nourished by the woman (according to the Aristotelian one-seed theory).[45] Massaria described the one-seed process of conception thus: 'in time of Copulation of the Male and Female, the Seed of the Male, is attracted into the Womb of the Female, and is extended, and dilated through all the parts thereof; and is there by the natural heat and moisture of the Womb, Coagulated into a massy substance'.[46] This massy substance then develops the various organs, leading 'if no mischance, or accident intervene to the hindrance thereof' to the birth of a child.[47] In order for reproduction to succeed, there should be no physiological defect to prevent the seed from reaching the womb, the body should be of the appropriate temperament to allow for the 'coagulation' to occur and finally the pregnancy should go through without any 'accidents'. Culpeper dedicated thirty pages of his *Directory for Midwives* to a list of the possible causes of barrenness in a couple, ranging from menstrual disorders and humoral distempers to lack of love between husband and wife.[48] In a later edition of Culpeper that was published posthumously, this list was followed by a briefer summary of those causes:

> All these causes are reduced either to Impotency in Copulation, or Distemper of the Stones and Seed Vessels, or evil Conformation, or a cold and moist distemper of the womb which cannot attract, detain and alter the seed. Sometimes a hot and dry distemper that cannot nourish the seed, or from the enlarging of the orifice after childbearing, or from humors, or being displaced, or the straitness of the vessels, or want of terms, or too many.[49]

The causes of infertility could thus be divided into two general categories: physical malformations and humoral imbalances known as 'distempers'. Physical malformations could prevent copulation entirely because of the shape or size of the sexual organs, or they could hinder the seed from reaching its destination even when copulation did occur. Because of their physical nature, many authors considered such malformations to be incurable, although some disagreed with this assessment. *The Expert Midwife* (1637), a translation of a text by the sixteenth-century Swiss physician Jacob Rueff, noted that 'barrennesse may be judged to proceed from the disposition and quality of the generative members . . . not a few infirmities and grievances doe happen to them, by reason of which man and wife are not onely made impotent and barren, but are unfit to dwell together'.[50] In this Rueff was following the legal distinction that a marriage which could not be consummated was not valid.[51] Massaria attributed to Hippocrates the claim that physical malformations were the principal cause of infertility, as in cases where 'the mouth of the Womb be ... turned aside out of its place, contrary from the *pudenda*, if the mouth of the Womb appear too big, or more wide than is convenient, or if the mouth of the womb be fallen down'.[52] Women whose bodies were malformed in this manner were deemed by Massaria 'unfit for conception', suggesting that such physical problems were indeed incurable.[53] Nicholas Fontanus was more forceful, stating that 'no physician can correct those errours which Nature commits in the mysterious purpose of our generation'. Fontanus was referring to 'errors' such as a cervix so narrow that it prevented proper ejaculation into the uterus as well as a cervix so wide that the seed immediately slips out after ejaculation.[54] By contrast, *The Compleat Midwives Practice* (1656) claimed that if barrenness was caused by 'the closing up of the Orifice of the womb', this 'may be cut and opened by Art'.[55] The idea that the womb could be 'closed' in a way that prevented the seed from reaching its destination was described poetically by Francois Mauriceau, who noted that it was 'not sufficient the Man's Yard enter the *vagina*, the Antichamber to the womb: for, if in the Act of Copulation, he knocks at the door, which is the internal orifice, and it not be opened, all is to no purpose'.[56]

It was understood that physical hindrances to conception prevented the seed from ever reaching the womb. Humoral explanations, meanwhile, centred on what happened to the seed once it arrived. A temperate womb with a moderate degree of heat and moisture was necessary for the process of 'coagulating' the seed and creating a child. Any extremes in the temperament of the womb could destroy the seed and cause infertility. To quote Fontanus: 'the temperate Matrix is most fruitfull, namely that which obtaines a mediocrity, approaching to no excesse'.[57] The seed, according to Fontanus, 'is a certain spirituall substance, generated of the purest part of the blood', and the delicate nature of the seed required that it 'should be concocted in a temperate womb; but if the *Matrix* be too hot, it consumes the seed, as a little water thrown into a fire, is presently dryed up'.[58] *Aristotle's Masterpiece* similarly claimed that excess heat corrupted the seed by drying it up, while excess cold made the seed 'waterish and unfit for generation'.[59] In addition to destroying the seed, an intemperate womb could also prevent the seed from reaching its destination in the first place. *The Compleat Midwives Practice* stated that infertility could be caused 'when the womb doth not attract the seed when it is cast in, which proceeds from a moist intemperance'.[60]

Massaria discussed conception using agricultural metaphors, in which the womb was the field in which the seed was planted. For him, a 'corrupt' field, or womb, was the most common cause of infertility in women. Like Fontanus, Massaria also considered excess heat and cold in the womb as causes of infertility, but he elaborated more on the matter of moisture, perhaps because this worked better with the agricultural theme. 'Immoderate moisture of the Womb,' he wrote, '. . . destroys the Seed of the man, as Corn sown in ponds and marshes.' 'Overmuch dryness', meanwhile, causes the seed to perish 'for want of nutriment, and [it] becomes as Corn sown upon stones, or sandy ground'.[61] Mary Fissell argues that early modern agricultural metaphors in which the male seed acted upon the female 'soil' privileged the role of men in the reproductive process, while reducing women to a more passive role. While the soil was important for providing nutrients and a place to grow, the active fertile potential lay in the seed. Fissell suggests that even when authors supported the two-seed model, they still privileged the male seed when describing conception in these terms.[62] When Jane Sharp used a similar metaphor to describe conception, she presented it in a way that made both partners active in the 'sowing' process, perhaps because of her unique position as a female midwife writing a midwifery manual. She wrote that 'True Conception is then, when the seed of both sexes is good, and duly prepared, and cast into the womb as into fruitful ground.'[63] However, Fissell's argument seems to discount the often active role given to the womb within midwifery manuals. The editor of Culpeper's posthumous edition stated that women were more often 'at fault' for infertility than men, because men's contribution to conception was much simpler than women's. Men's bodies only needed to provide 'fruitful seed spent into a fruitful womb', whereas women 'besides the meeting of their own seed, must receive, retain and nourish the man's, and afford matter for the forming of the child, in which divers accidents happen, and any of these will cause Barrenness'.[64] The role of the woman's body here seems more active than Fissell's interpretation suggests. The womb does not simply serve as a passive 'soil' in which the seed is planted, but must also actively receive or even suck in the male seed, add its own seed to it and then close up in order to retain the seed within it.

Menstrual disorders could also be related to problems in conception, although this was not the only context in which they were understood. Lisa Smith points out that the absence of menstruation was not automatically understood as a sign of pregnancy or a form of fertility problem, but rather as a general sign of ill health or a blockage in the body.[65] Nonetheless, early modern people also recognized the link between menstruation and fertility. They also believed that an excess of menstrual fluid, or menstrual blood of a specific colour or quality, could cause infertility. These were humoral disorders, because blood was one of the four humours and menstrual blood was part of the larger economy of humours in the body.[66] If it did not flow in an appropriate manner, this indicated a humoral imbalance. The link between menstrual blood and the broader economy of the humours can be seen in the claim made by Culpeper that 'A third cause of Natural Barrenness is the letting of Virgin's blood in the Arm before their courses come down', suggesting that the letting of regular blood could prevent the proper function of menstrual blood.[67] Any 'obstruction in the flowers', as *The Compleat Midwives Practice* put it, could cause infertility.[68] Massaria listed menstruation among the necessary factors to ensure conception. He claimed that 'the monethly Terms are greatly to be respected, as hinderers or furtherers thereof [of fertility]; if they come not in due order, it must necessarily cause barrenness of that woman to follow'.[69] Menstrual disorders could also be caused by physical factors, such as an excessively narrow cervix that prevented the flow. This form of amenorrhoea caused a humoral imbalance in the body, thus not only preventing conception but also 'bring[ing] forth many other evils'.[70]

Although the common belief was that 'barrenness is oftener from a fault in the women than the men',[71] manuals did discuss male fertility problems, which were not limited to impotence or even to physical deformities in the penis. Like women, men's fertility problems could stem from deformities that prevented copulation or hindered the proper ejaculation of the seed, or they could arise from humoral distempers that caused the seed to fail in its purpose despite entering the womb.[72] It was important for a man to be 'furnished with fit instruments', specifically 'the yard, stones and seed', as well as that he be able to copulate.[73] It seems self-evident that a man without a functioning penis or testes (which were understood to be the location where male seed was 'concocted') would be unable to impregnate his wife, and a man with a missing penis or testicles might very well have been prevented from marrying at all.[74] Physical deformities in the penis were a less obvious cause of male infertility, 'as if the same [the penis] be oblique or crooked, if any of the ligaments thereof be distorted, or broken, whereby the wayes and passages through which the seed should flow be corrupt, stopped or vituated'.[75]

The requirement for 'fit seed' is more significant, because it demonstrates that early modern physicians recognized that a man could be fully capable of performing sexually and even having his seed reach the womb, but still fail to produce children. The quality of the man's seed was of crucial importance because the male seed was considered the active conveyor of fertility. This was certainly true for those who adhered to a 'one-seed' model in which only men had seed which was 'sown' in the womb. However, even those who adhered to a 'two-seed' model believed that the male seed played a more important role in the reproductive process. Sharp noted that 'the seed of the Male is more active than that of the Female in forming the creature, though both be fruitful', and Helkiah Crooke claimed that 'the seed of a man is the active principle of the body, that of the women but the passive, or at least far lesse active than the other'.[76] Like menstrual blood, the male seed was part of the humoral economy of the body and was believed to be concocted out of blood. Thus the seed could fail in its purpose because it was of an improper temperament. It is important to note that when Culpeper or Massaria discussed the need for a 'fit' or 'fruitful' seed, they were not simply referring to a man's ability to visibly ejaculate. Although early modern medicine did not explicitly differentiate between semen and sperm, there are indications that they acknowledged that cases existed in which a man's seed was successfully 'cast forth' but was 'vitious and unfit for generation'.[77] Here the temperament of the seed itself caused the problem, rather than any failure to produce it.[78]

Physical Moderation

Humoral imbalances were either behavioural or they were inherent to the patient's temperament and nature. This meant that a patient who was diagnosed with a humoral imbalance was subject to overt and implied criticism regarding their morality and adherence to social norms. The balance of humours in the body was affected by a variety of lifestyle factors. Diet, exercise, sexual behaviour and even emotions such as anger were all believed to affect the body and create distempers which could hinder reproduction. These were all factors that carried moral and religious judgements. Proper early modern men and women were expected to avoid lust, gluttony, idleness and wrath, and to conduct themselves in modesty and moderation.[79] These were factors that patients could ostensibly control and alter, so that when midwifery manuals argued that specific behaviours caused infertility, they invited their readers to re-examine their lives and consider whether something in their own conduct contributed to their problem.

Given the link between sexual activity and reproduction, it is hardly surprising that information about proper sexual conduct had a central place in midwifery manuals. Following the principle of moderation, manuals advised against overly frequent copulation or infrequent copulation. Fontanus stated that 'if it [infertility] arise from frequent coition, the incontinent person must curb her, or his appetites'.[80] No details were given as to what constituted 'too much' activity. This common-sense advice is still given to couples wishing to conceive today, but in the early modern period this was accompanied by the moral weight of beliefs about sexuality and about gendered expectations regarding sexual conduct. Women were believed to be lustful and to have greater difficulty in controlling their sexual urges, yet good women were expected to be chaste, faithful and obedient to their husbands. Women were at once more susceptible to sexual immorality and more censured when they succumbed to it.[81] The association between coldness and asexuality has been preserved in the English language through the use of the word 'frigid' to describe women who have no sexual desire. The word was first used to describe someone lacking in sexual vigour in 1660, but it did not become particularly associated with women until the early twentieth century.[82] In the humoral system, women were expected to be colder than men, although an excess of cold prevented them from fulfilling their womanly role by becoming mothers. Excess heat in women was more complicated in terms of gender identity, because heat was a quality that was associated with men and encapsulated their strength, vigour and action. A woman who was overly hot was therefore also overly masculine, her body physically transgressing proper gender boundaries and becoming infertile as a result. When midwifery manuals associated excessive heat in women with sexual lust and licence, they also suggested that this excess masculinity made a woman less able to moderate her behaviour and act as a demure and chaste matron. Although men were considered more 'perfect' than women because of their heat, women who were excessively hot were not understood as better women but as unwomanly. Rueff noted that women 'which are over man-like, are not so apt for generation', nor are men 'which are more effeminate and woman-like than is requisite'.[83] For women excess manliness caused irregular menstruation, while for men effeminacy was related to a cold and moist distemper, making them unable to produce fertile seed.

The early modern concern with women's lust on the one hand, and the requirement that they be chaste and loyal to their husbands on the other, meant that midwifery manuals tended to be more forgiving towards sexual excesses from men than from women, although both were believed to hinder fertility. Fontanus claimed that women who had 'plentiful courses' were both more likely to be fertile and more sexual, but he did not give much detail about the positive, fertility-promoting aspects of female sexuality. Instead he censured women's lustfulness and promiscuity by linking it unequivocally with infertility. He wrote:

> Other sorts of barren women must be referred to [in] this Catalogue as those that are luxuriant [tending to excess], and the whorish crew; the former, because by frequent coition their bodies become empty of seed, and if any at that time be ejaculated, it is not fit for generation... and the latter sort conceive not... partly by reason of their frequent cohabitation with men, whereby the neck of the Matrix is made so slippery that it cannot release the man's seed.[84]

Fontanus believed that an excess of sexual activity in a woman, whether she was a prostitute or merely promiscuous, would cause her seed to fail and her womb to reject a man's seed.[85] He was writing within a medical context, but was using this medical context to engage with a broader world view. Women were believed to be inherently over-sexual and Fontanus claimed that women were required to control this sexual excess if they wanted to conceive. Other authors had similar views about the links between excessive female sexuality and infertility. Massaria claimed that women who were barren owing to excessive heat were 'hasty and Chollerick, quick witted and crafty, thirsty and desirous after carnall copulation'.[86] *Aristotle's Masterpiece* differentiated between hot women and cold women, stating that women who were barren because of excess heat 'love to play in the courts of Venus', while women who were barren owing to coldness were the exact opposite.[87]

Male sexual licence was treated more forgivingly, as virile men were expected to perform sexually and desire sex.[88] However, self-control was also a part of masculine expression in this period, and too much sexual activity on the part of a man could result in the loss of his masculine heat, causing him not only to become infertile but also to become weak and emasculated.[89] Male sexuality was a sign of a healthy body and temperament. Fertile men were 'cheerefull, affable, ever frequenting the young company of Maids, and Virgins, being excited by the flagrancy of their eyes to *Venereous* dalliances and lustfull speculations', but infertile men were not lacking in sexual desire. They were more 'desirous of venery, than able to performe it'.[90] An excess of sexual appetite and activity in a man could lead to an unhealthy and weakened state. 'Those that use immoderate Copulation', wrote Massaria, 'are very weak in their bodies, seeing the whole body is thereby deprived of its best & purest blood & of the vital spirits.'[91] This in turn could lead them to fail in performing their reproductive duties. 'Too frequent carnal Copulation, is one great cause of barrenness of men,' Massaria continued, because it 'attracteth the seminal moisture from the stones, before it is sufficiently prepared and concocted'.[92]

Sexual moderation was important to reproduction, but it was not the only behavioural factor that influenced fertility. Both men and women were advised to avoid extremes in food, drink, activity and emotions in order to conceive. These factors corresponded to the sins of lust, gluttony, idleness and wrath. By connecting these social and spiritual transgressions with the needs of the reproducing body, medical authors reinforced social norms by tying them to the physical world and linking them to earthly consequences. They also drew from the Classical medical tradition and operated within the internal logic of humoral medicine. The social and the medical were inextricably linked. Moreover, the behaviours that triggered infertility were also linked to the idle wealthy, so that medical advice also became a form of social commentary, criticizing the lifestyle of the immoderate elites. Sarah Toulalan suggests that excessive eating or fatness were qualities more likely to be associated with the wealthy, and these were indeed linked to infertility.[93] Massaria noted that 'Glutony and drunkenness do also much hinder men from fruitfulness'.[94] James Wolveridge advised women against 'too great hunger; for by overmuch fulness the infant is sooner suffocated, the passages appointed for nourishment being the sooner obstructed'.[95] Nicholas Culpeper similarly tied infertility to idleness, and connected it explicitly with the inactivity of upper class city women, which he considered sinful. He suggested that women who wanted to conceive should 'give themselves to exercise. Idleness is hateful to God and destructive to creation, and that's the reason such women as live idly, (as more of our City Dames do) have so few children, and those they have seldom live.'[96] Other authors did not make the link quite so explicitly, but they also cautioned against excessive inactivity. Wolveridge listed 'overmuch sleep, and a continuall laziness' as causes of miscarriage, and *The Compleat Midwives Practice* listed 'much sleep' as causing the womb to 'not draw the seed which is ejected'.[97] Sharp further highlighted the significance of moderation in activity, stating that 'nothing furthers good concoction more than moderate labour, for it stirs up natural heat; whereas idle persons breed crude humours'.[98]

While idleness was one source of concern, women were also cautioned against an excess of activity, particularly of a kind that was perhaps inappropriate for matrons, such as running, leaping and dancing.[99] Such views did not remain on the theoretical level, as Chapter 2 demonstrated. When James II criticized his daughter Mary for her lack of care during pregnancy, leading in his opinion to miscarriage, or when Charles I assured his mother-in-law that her daughter would be more careful in her next pregnancy, they were echoing these views.[100] These were then used to control what women could do during pregnancy and also to hold them accountable for the success or failure of their own reproductive endeavours.

Emotional Control

The moderation of appetites, sexual and otherwise, was tied to religious morality and to cultural perceptions about how men and women ought to behave. Advice about emotional moderation went deeper, to fundamental views about the gendered order and the place of women and men within it. Statements about the importance of love and affection in marriage served to reinforce ideas about the family, the most basic social unit in early modern society. At the same time, statements about the impact of hatred or anger on fertility served to remind women of their place within marriage, and to remind them of the significance of quiet obedience to the fulfilment of their wifely duties. If women were advised that anger would hinder their fertility, this served to reinforce the idea that wives should not express outright anger at their husbands.[101] Gail Kern Paster argues that by cautioning pregnant women against excessive anger and other emotions, Culpeper, Guillameu and others were using physiology 'to reinforce a conventional construction of the female body . . . and to contest the social privilege that pregnancy gave to the mother-to-be to 'have her longing'.[102] In other words, pregnant women were denied any special rights accorded to their status, through the indication that they might be endangering the pregnancy. Extreme anger and extreme sorrow were believed to prevent conception, according to *The Compleat Midwife*, and 'sudden fury, great wrath, over much fear and sorrow, sudden joy' were all potential causes of miscarriage.[103] In her study of women's anger in early modern England, Gwynne Kennedy also notes that female anger was understood as a cause of amenorrhoea and as a danger to the proper formation of the foetus.[104]

While admonitions regarding the impact of anger on conception and pregnancy served to constrain and limit women, they also acted to reinforce other ideologies. In principle, early modern men ruled their household and they held authority over their wives, but the properly masculine management of the household demanded that they do so with moderation and through respect and love. If they resorted instead to violence or fear, they seemingly lost some of their 'proper' control.[105] Therefore, pregnant women were given some power when dealing with their husbands and male authorities because of the idea that if men caused their wives anger or sorrow they risked the family's chances of reproduction.[106] At the same time, this also served as a reminder to women of their place in the social order. Adrian Wilson argues strongly against an unnuanced presentation of the ideal of 'obedience' within early modern marriage and of the husband's authority over his wife. He argues that

> there was simply no means at all for enforcing the wife's vow to 'obey and serve' her husband. Ironically, therefore, the husband's authority – enshrined in the marriage-service, affirmed in the common law, bound up with coverture and thus linked with the juridical inequality of the sexes – rested on the flimsiest of foundations.[107]

Wilson's call for nuance is an important reminder, and he suggests that ultimately the husband's authority stemmed from the wife's willingness to give him that authority by fulfilling the duty of obedience. If this was the case, however, then when midwifery manuals cautioned women that anger or improper behaviours would hinder their fertility, they were doing more than just echoing general 'gendered norms'. They were shoring up the 'flimsy foundation' on which the ideal of obedience stood, by arguing that fertility itself depended on the fulfilment of wifely duties.

What was true regarding anger as a negative force within marriage was also true for love and affection as positive forces. According to William Gouge, author of one of the most influential treatises on marital life in the seventeenth century, couples should 'mutually delight each in other, and maintaine a pure and fervent love betwixt themselves'.[108] Gouge also argued that 'a loving mutuall affection must passe betwixt husband and wife, or else no dutie will be well performed: this is the ground of all the rest'.[109] Other authors of medical guides also included both sexual relations and love in their ideology of marriage, although they differed on the precise meaning of this love and the place it had within marital power relations.[110] The view of marriage as an institution based on consent and mutual affection was fundamental to the understanding of conception and fertility, because childbearing was a central part of early modern marriage. According to midwifery manuals, a fruitful marriage would have to meet several requirements, which closely echoed the outlines of a good marriage laid down by Gouge and others.[111] Simply put, the manuals stated that for conception to occur: (a) both men and women had to enjoy the sexual act, (b) both the sexual act and the marriage had to be consensual, and (c) the marriage had to be loving and affectionate. A lack in any of these things could cause the match to be infertile. These claims were all nominally explained by humoral theory, but they were also closely linked to cultural and religious views of the ideal marriage.

Numerous historians of early modern reproduction have focused on the claim that sexual pleasure was necessary for conception, and in particular on Thomas Laqueur's argument that the necessity of female orgasm for conception was the defining characteristic of pre-Enlightenment views of the body.[112] While midwifery manuals did imply that female orgasm was necessary for conception, focusing on that as the *central* requirement ignores the broader terms in which manuals discussed sexual pleasure. It also marginalizes the emphasis manual writers put on other aspects of marital life, namely consent, love and affection. Certainly, in some cases manuals did describe the necessity of a sexual peak that can be understood as an orgasm. In *The Practice of Physick* (1655) Lazarus Riverius suggested that infertility was caused because 'the Woman being averse from this kind of pleasure, [she] gives not down [a] sufficient quantity of Spirits, wherewith her Genitals ought to swell at the instant of Generation, that her womb skipping as it were for joy, may meet her Husband's sperm . . . and draw it into its innermost Cavity . . . and sprinkle it with her own Sperm, powr'd forth in that pang of Pleasure . . . '.[113] It is difficult to read this passage without seeing it as a reference to female orgasm, or indeed mutual orgasm. Other manuals also argued that women must enjoy the sexual act in order to conceive, but they used terms that were far broader, such as pleasure, contentment or desire. A women might be barren if she 'perceives very little or no pleasure in the act of copulation', but if 'after she hath had the company of her husband she hath received more content than ordinary', this was a sign that she conceived.[114] An infertile couple was one that comes 'to the school of Venus . . . so coldly that as good never a whit'.[115] Even Fontanus, who claimed dismissively that sexual pleasure 'condueceth little or nothing to conception', nonetheless stated that women do 'enjoy unspeakable pleasure' when they conceive.[116] Female sexual pleasure was necessary for conception in both the 'one-seed' and 'two-seed' models of reproduction. In the 'two-seed' model it was necessary for the woman to release her own seed, while in both models pleasure played a crucial role in preparing the womb to accept sperm. When a woman took pleasure in copulation, 'the womb being covetous of the Seed, opens itself to receive it'.[117] If the womb failed to open, 'the most frequent reason' was 'the insensibility of some women, who take no pleasure in the venereal act'.[118] The womb played quite an active role in early modern midwifery manuals, expected to open up and draw or suck the sperm into its depth.[119] As Jennifer Evans demonstrates, the importance of male and female sexual pleasure to conception meant that aphrodisiacs, used to promote both the sexual act itself and its enjoyment, were often part of the treatment of fertility problems.[120]

The importance of sexual pleasure for conception was in accordance with the mainstream view that providing mutual pleasure was one of the duties of married couples, even when it was not meant for procreation. This meant that conception was supposed to be enjoyable, not merely a formal duty.[121] This ideology was embodied by medical beliefs that claimed that not only were both members of the couple expected to enjoy the sexual act, but that both parties were required to consent to it, and to marriage itself, in order to reproduce successfully. If parents forced their children to marry against their will, this might cause the marriage to be infertile. The medical explanation for this requirement was that a person's emotional state could influence the proper function of the body. 'Extream hatred', Jane Sharp claimed, 'is the reason why women seldom or never conceive when they are ravished.' Married couples could also hate each other to a degree that causes infertility, 'commonly when they are contracted and married by unkind Parents for some sinister ends against their wills'.[122] *Aristotle's Masterpiece* similarly argued for the importance of consensual marriage to successful reproduction. When parents forced their children to marry, they married 'their bodies, but not their hearts, and where there is want of Love, there for the most part is no Conception'.[123] Most marriages in the early modern period were fertile. Most of them were also not romantic marriages in the modern sense. Instead most marriages were neither a simple marriage by choice, nor a forced marriage, but rather the result of a process of selection and negotiation in which couples, family and kin acted together in order to decide on a match.[124] The stress that midwifery manuals placed on consensual marriage as a necessity for conception indicates that most marriages were seen as, in some sense, consensual. Consent was also a legal and religious requirement for marriage in this period.[125] It was almost unacceptable to outright force a couple to marry, and when the authors of manuals stated, often quite strongly, that such a union could not be fertile, they were turning social norm into physical fact, echoing and reinforcing cultural ideology. This link between the social and the medical is most clearly evident in Culpeper's warning that infertility was caused by 'that trick of Parents to compel their Children to marry against their minds. Such corrupt beginnings usually bring forth sorrow enough to all parties.'[126]

If hatred could prevent conception, then love promoted it. Phillip Barrough, author of one of the earliest popular medical guides in English, *The Method of Physick* (1583), stated plainly that 'love causeth conception'.[127] Although not referring to modern conceptions of romantic love, early modern marital ideology did encourage affection and attachment between spouses. Midwifery manuals reinforced this idea by stating that love was a necessary component for conception even when they did not provide any medical logic for it. The editor of the posthumous edition of Culpeper's *Directory* admonished couples to avoid anger, sadness and fear during copulation, if they wanted to conceive, and instead 'let love be invited, and if it burn, there will many Spirits flie to the womb and privities'.[128] In this case love seems to act as a magnet for some humoral substance (the spirits), drawing them into the womb and assisting conception.[129] In other cases, however, love's role was understood more as a kind of sympathetic magic. If people hated each other, their bodies would reject one another and would therefore not combine in order to create new life. If they loved each other, the seeds would be drawn to each other, or the seed to the womb. As Culpeper put it, 'If their hearts not be united in love, how should their seed unite to cause conception?'[130]

The argument that anger, hatred or even an excessive tendency to vices would cause infertility was one that had abundant evidence to the contrary. Anne Dormer was trapped in a miserable marriage with an abusive husband whose death in 1689 brought her nothing but relief. They had eleven children. Her sister, Elizabeth Trumbull, was married for thirty-four years to a man she loved dearly, and whose attachment to her shows in every one of the dozens of letters he wrote to her. The couple was childless.[131] While the contrast between the two sisters is particularly powerful, it could hardly be unusual that an unhappy marriage was fruitful or a happy one infertile. Presumably there were also many drunkards who fathered children, and prostitutes were quite clearly not universally childless.[132] Yet midwifery manuals repeatedly made these claims even when they were not commensurate with experience. The most obvious challenge to these concepts was conception as a result of rape. Jane Sharp and the author of *Aristotle's Masterpiece* both claimed that it was unusual for rape to end in pregnancy, precisely because of the necessity of love and consent.[133] Theoretically, if a woman was pregnant, it followed that she had not been raped. Yet even in the seventeenth century legal realities did not conform to these medical views, and rape cases were not automatically dismissed on the grounds that the victim was pregnant. One method of resolving this conflict was by arguing that it was possible for the mind to deny consent, while the body still took pleasure in the sexual act sufficiently to conceive. The act could then be deemed rape, despite the pregnancy.[134] Such creative thinking indicates an awareness of some tension between the theory of conception as it was promoted by medical writers and the practice of conception in the real world.

How could early modern readers resolve these tensions, and make sense of the potential contradictions between the theoretical causes of infertility and their lived experiences? Perhaps they didn't need to. Early modern concepts of truth and evidence did not function as modern scientific views dictate. When it came to early modern medicine, and in particular women's bodies, various complex and ambiguous concepts coexisted without being perceived as contradictory. Early modern medical interpretations of nature were fairly relaxed and allowed some leeway for the 'preternatural', those things that were at the extreme or the contradiction of natural rule, yet were seen as part of nature.[135] Such preternatural things were increasingly understood less as potentially supernatural or miraculous, and more as 'almost-natural'.[136] The idea that natural laws were not immutable but rather general rules, together with the idea of the preternatural as something that deviated somewhat from the natural order, but did not destroy it, allowed the early modern mind to accept that certain things were natural laws even when there were obvious contradictions to them. So medical writers could present love or consent as necessary elements of conception, and at the same time account for any cases in which conception occurred without them. This was further made possible by the very nature of Galenic humoral medicine, which tied each medical diagnosis to the specific situation of the specific body rather than to any general description, so that any deviation from the general rules might be explained by some specific temperament or condition.[137]

Magical Explanations

Infertility was usually understood as having natural causes, and in some cases these may have skirted on the preternatural; but one final explanatory model for infertility lay firmly within the realm of the supernatural. This was the recurring claim in medical manuals that infertility might be caused by magic or witchcraft. Those who made this claim were somewhat cautious about it, because it had the uncomfortable implication that witchcraft might go against God's own plan, but it nonetheless appeared in several contexts.[138] The presence of supernatural explanations of infertility within medical texts serves not only as a reminder of the enduring power of demonic beliefs in early modern England, but also of the elision between medicine, religion and magic in this period.[139] The physician and apothecary William Drage dedicated his 1614 treatise *Daimonomageia* to those sicknesses and diseases which were caused by witchcraft. According to Drage, 'Diseases that are caused by Nature, may be caused by Witchcraft. But all that are caused by Witchcraft cannot be caused by Nature.' Among the diseases caused by witchcraft he included barrenness, sterility and impotence.[140] Midwifery manuals also listed witchcraft as a cause of infertility. 'If the party be bewitched,' advised Fontanus, 'besides the ordinary helps, you must indeavor to subdue the evill with other means . . . for some diseases and remedies exceed the limits and boundaries of Nature.'[141] 'It is not one Physitians opinion alone that many Women are made Barren by diabolical means,' Culpeper noted, but following his faith he took care to indicate that by this he meant 'an abuse of Nature' rather than specifically the invocation of evil spirits.[142] Jakob Rueff, *The Compleat Midwife*, Nicholas Sudell and Jane Sharp also specified that barrenness could be caused by enchantment.[143] Authors of midwifery manuals, both those translated from Continental sources and those written in English, recognized witchcraft as a cause of infertility that was 'unnatural' and outside the purview of medicine. If they suggested any means of curing such infertility, these were magical means, such as urinating through a wedding ring.[144] These cures were part of a long tradition of magical and semi-magical cures for fertility problems, prevalent in Europe.[145]

The frequent reference to witchcraft as a cause of infertility is intriguing, because infertility makes almost no appearance in actual English witchcraft cases. There is evidence that magical practices were used to promote fertility, and it also seems very likely that among practitioners of folk magic there was some use of magic to prevent conception or cause miscarriage, both for contraceptive reasons and in order to harm other women.[146] However, this form of magic made little appearance in official records of English witchcraft. The only case I have found in which a witch explicitly prevented a couple from conceiving was that of the family of Francis Manners, Earl of Rutland, dating from 1618.[147] The case centred on Joan Flower and her two daughters, who had been in the employ of the earl or living in his household. The countess took some dislike to one of the daughters, Margaret, and dismissed her from the house, giving her some pay in compensation. Soon afterwards, the earl failed to take Joan's side in a dispute with another of his employees. According to Margaret's confession, these two matters caused her to hold a grudge against the countess and the earl and to plot her revenge against them. According to the case record, Margaret, her mother and her sister Phillip [*sic*] used witchcraft in order to kill the Rutlands' children and to prevent the couple from having any others, possibly by causing the countess to miscarry. In her examination Margaret admitted that they had plotted against the Rutlands 'that they might have no more children'. They did this by taking a pair of gloves, dipping them in water, mixing them with blood and then rubbing them on the belly of their cat, Rutterkin. Margaret claimed that this would not render the Rutlands permanently infertile, but would delay conception.[148] The case also made an appearance in a ballad entitled *The Damnable Practices of Three Lincolne-shire witches* (1619). The bulk of the ballad discussed the ways in which the witches tormented the Rutlands and killed their living children. There is only a brief mention of the conspiracy to prevent them from having any additional offspring:

> And likewise she [Margaret] confessed how they,
> Together all agreed;
> Against the children of this Earle,
> To practice and proceed,
> Not leaving them a child alive,

And never to have more,
If witchcraft so could doe, because,
They turned them [the Flowers] out of dore.[149]

The main focus of the accusation against the Flowers witches was that of trying to leave the Rutlands childless through witchcraft. The primary harm was done by killing all their existing children, and preventing additional births was only the last step of this process. Causing infertility can be seen as an extension of the more typical child-murdering accusation which was often levelled against witches, rather than a case in which the witches' main purpose was to cause infertility.[150]

Some witches were accused of causing miscarriages or of harming or attempting to harm a child while it was still in its mother's womb. Again, these were extensions of the usual child-murder accusations, rather than a reference to uniquely reproductive magic. In 1650 Margaret White of Northumberland confessed that she and her accomplices tried to use witchcraft to 'consume the child' that was in the womb of a Mrs Moore, but that 'the Lord would not permit' this to happen. They had to wait until after the child was born in order to harm it.[151] It is interesting that God's protection over an unborn child seemed stronger than the protection afforded to an infant. Another woman, Jannet Hargrave, was accused of killing a child in the belly of Ellen Robinson in an undated case.[152] These rare cases do not make up any significant trend within English witchcraft cases. The rarity may be the result of the contingencies of English witchcraft laws, which legislated against causing particular harm (*maleficia*) through witchcraft rather than against witchcraft as such.[153] Demonstrating that a child had been killed or a woman taken ill was one thing, but demonstrating that someone had been made unable to have children was rather more difficult. It is therefore possible that magic was used in order to hinder or promote fertility, but the inability to demonstrate specific *maleficia* prevented it from reaching trial.

There is some indication that certain forms of magic, rather than deliberate and demonic acts of witchcraft, were understood as causing infertility. Nicholas Culpeper listed several 'external causes' for infertility which can be understood as magical causes rather than medical ones, because they did not operate within a humoral logic but rather relied on sympathetic relations or other magical methods that often did not involve any contact with the body. Culpeper indicated that hanging a hart's tongue near the bed would cause infertility, a cause that clearly did not operate within normal humoral parameters. A woman walking over another woman's 'terms' could also cause infertility, a magical act that followed the rules of sympathetic magic, with one woman's menses affecting another woman's fertility.[154] One mid-seventeenth-century collection of magical charms and spells listed a potion to make a woman infertile, utilizing 'The barke of white poplar drunke with the kidney of a mule'.[155] The mule, as a barren animal, could trigger infertility in a woman. Interestingly, this is one of the only recipes in this text to be written in English rather than Latin, the more typical language of learned magical treatises. It seems unlikely that a woman could accidentally step over another's menstrual blood or ingest a drink made of the kidney of mule without knowing she had done so. This suggests that perhaps such spells were meant to be used more as contraceptive magic than as a malicious means of causing infertility in another. Their existence does suggest that some magical means of causing sterility were recognized in England.

The rarity of English witchcraft cases related to causing infertility begs the question of why enchantment appeared repeatedly in English midwifery manuals as a cause of infertility. One possible explanation may lie in the way medical knowledge was transmitted across Europe. If fertility played a more central role in Continental witchcraft cases, as Lyndal Roper argues, it may have appeared frequently in Continental midwifery manuals.[156] These ideas may have made their way into English manuals by way of the many translations of Continental texts, from which they were copied or edited into manuals written by English authors. In his ground-breaking work on beliefs about pregnancy and fertility in early modern France, Jacques Gélis highlights the abundance of magical and semi-magical beliefs surrounding infertility in this period. He notes that while infertility was usually considered physiological, 'unnatural or magical practices were also sometimes suspected', and notes numerous curative practices relating to water, trees and stones.[157] Early modern England was home to communities of Continental immigrants, who may have brought their own beliefs about magic and witchcraft with them to England, including those relating to the causes of infertility.[158] Mentions of witchcraft may also have been meant as sources of titillation, adding another selling point to books that were already on the border between practical manuals and exciting sex guides.[159] Despite the rarity of fertility-related cases in English witchcraft cases, the prevalence of mentions of magic and witchcraft as causes of infertility in midwifery manuals suggests that such beliefs were relatively widespread. At the very least it was not incongruous for a medical writer to suggest that witches could cause direct harm to the proper function of the body, even in the late seventeenth century.

Conclusion

An early modern couple who sought an explanation for their fertility problem did not have to look far. A wide range of popular medical manuals offered clear explanations for difficulties in conception, miscarriages and other reproductive disorders. Such a couple would, however, be faced with a holistic medical view that forced them to examine their lives and consider whether personality flaws or their own misconduct caused them to be infertile. The religious belief that infertility was a punishment of sins or a test of faith found reinforcement in medical manuals that suggested infertility was caused by promiscuity, gluttony, idleness or transgressions of proper gendered behaviours such as excessive masculinity in a woman or effeminacy in a man. This is not to state that medical texts did not provide a clear and coherent medical view. They placed the causes of infertility firmly within the humoral framework, provided some diagnostic methods for identifying whether the problem lay with the husband or the wife, and offered a wealth of advice on treating fertility problems once they were diagnosed. Midwifery manuals were practical guides to conception and childbirth, and their popularity and the evidence that they were used indicates that patients found them useful. They were at once practical medical guides and comportment manuals that promoted religious and social views about proper conduct, marital life and gendered behaviour. Medical explanations of infertility were not parallel to or competing with religious or even magical views of the problem, but rather highlight the elision of the three views.

Notes

1. Eucharius Roesslin, *The Byrth of Mankynde Newly Translated Out of Laten into Englysshe, Etc.* (London: Thomas Raynalde, 1540), pp. LXXXI–LXXXIV.
2. Mary Whitelocke, *Advice for Her Son Samuel*, Princeton University RTC01 Ms. 226, unnumbered.
3. Whitelocke, *Advice for Her Son Samuel.*
4. Alexandra Walsham, *Providence in Early Modern England* (Oxford: Oxford University Press, 1999), pp. 2–3.

5. Walsham, *Providence in Early Modern England*, 13, 16. Andrew Wear, *Knowledge and Practice in English Medicine, 1550–1680* (Cambridge: Cambridge University Press, 2000), pp. 30–31.
6. Charles Gibbon, *A Vvork Vvorth the Reading* (London: Imprinted by Thomas Orwin, 1591), p. 17. John Hacket, *A Century of Sermons Upon Several Remarkable Subjects Preached by the Right Reverend Father in God, John Hacket* (London: Printed by Andrew Clark for Robert Scott, 1675), p. 80.
7. Edmund Grindal, *A Sermon, at the Funeral Solemnitie of the Most High and Mighty Prince Ferdinandus* (London: By Iohn Day, 1564), unnumbered.
8. Donald Lupton, *Obiectorum Reductio: Or, Daily Imployment for the Soule* (London: Printed by Iohn Norton, for Iohn Rothwell 1634), p. 55. 'The woman's body is the terrain on which patriarchy is erected', Adrienne Rich, *Of Woman Born: Motherhood as Experience and Institution*, (New York: Norton, 1995), p. 55.
9. Lisa W. Smith, 'La Raillerie Des Femmes? Les Femmes, La Stérilité Et La Société En France a L'époque Moderne', in *Femmes En Fleurs, Femmes En Corps: Sang, Santé, Sexualités Du Moyen Age Aux Lumières*, ed. Cathy McClive and Nicole Pellegrin (Saint-Étienne: Publications de l'Université de Saint-Étienne, 2010), pp. 203–220.
10. Ian Maclean, 'Evidence, Logic, the Rule and the Exception in Renaissance Law and Medicine', *Early Science and Medicine* 5, no. 3 (2000): 23n.
11. Elizabeth A. Foyster, *Manhood in Early Modern England: Honour, Sex, and Marriage* (London: Longman, 1999), p. 76.
12. Richard Newhauser, '"These Seaven Devils": The Capital Vices on the Way to Modernity', in *Sin in Medieval and Early Modern Culture: The Tradition of the Seven Deadly Sins*, ed. Richard Newhauser and Susan Janet Ridyard (York: York Medieval Press, 2012).
13. David Harley, 'Spiritual Physic, Providence and English Medicine, 1560–1640', in *Medicine and the Reformation*, ed. Ole Peter Grell and Andrew Cunningham (London, New York: Routledge, 1993). Karen Harvey, 'The History of Masculinity, Circa 1650–1800', *The Journal of British Studies* 44, no. 2 (2005): 296–311.
14. Todd W. Reeser, *Moderating Masculinity in Early Modern Culture* (Chapel Hill: University of North Carolina Press, 2006), p. 13.
15. Ethan H. Shagan, *The Rule of Moderation: Violence, Religion and the Politics of Restraint in Early Modern England* (Cambridge: Cambridge University Press, 2011), p. 8.
16. Lisa W. Smith, 'Imagining Women's Fertility Before Technology', *Journal of Medical Humanities* 31, no. 1 (2010): 77.
17. Laura Gowing, *Gender Relations in Early Modern England* (Harlow: Pearson Education, 2012), p. 8.

18. Susanne Scholz, *Body Narratives: Writing the Nation and Fashioning the Subject in Early Modern England* (Basingstoke: Palgrave Macmillan, 2000), p. 16.
19. Mary Fissell, 'Gender and Generation: Representing Reproduction in Early Modern England', *Gender & History* 7, no. 3 (1995): 434.
20. Harley, 'Spiritual Physic, Providence and English Medicine, 1560–1640'.
21. Mary Lindemann, *Medicine and Society in Early Modern Europe* (Cambridge: Cambridge University Press, 2010), p. 13. Smith, 'Imagining Women's Fertility before Technology', 70.
22. Angus McLaren, *Reproductive Rituals: The Perception of Fertility in England from the Sixteenth to the Nineteenth Century* (London: Methuen, 1984), pp. 33–35.
23. Hippocrates, *The Aphorisms of Hippocrates: With a Translation into Latin and English* (London: A. J. Valpy, 1822), p. 150.
24. William Harvey, *Anatomical Exercitations Concerning the Generation of Living Creatures* (London: Printed by James Young for Octavian Pulleyn, 1653). Sarah Toulalan, '"Elderly Years Cause a Total Dispaire of Conception": Old Age, Sex and Infertility in Early Modern England', *Social History of Medicine* 29, no. 2 (2016): 333–359. Alexander Massaria, *Prælectiones De Morbis Mulierum, Conceptus Et Partus* (Lipsiæ, 1600).
25. Audrey Eccles, *Obstetrics and Gynaecology in Tudor and Stuart England* (Kent, OH: Kent State University Press, 1982), pp. 11–15.
26. Eccles, *Obstetrics and Gynaecology in Tudor and Stuart England*, 11–15. Mary Fissell, *Vernacular Bodies: The Politics of Reproduction in Early Modern England* (Oxford: Oxford University Press, 2004). Mary Fissell, 'Making a Masterpiece: The Aristotle Texts in Vernacular Medical Culture', in *Right Living: An Anglo-American Tradition of Self-Help Medicine and Hygiene*, ed. C.E. Rosenberg (Baltimore, MD: Johns Hopkins University Press, 2003).
27. Trotula, *Medieval Woman's Guide to Health: The First English Gynecological Handbook* (Kent, OH: Kent State University Press, 1981).
28. Edith L. Klotz, 'A Subject Analysis of English Imprints for Every Tenth Year from 1480 to 1640', *Huntington Library Quarterly* 1, no. 4 (1938): 417–419.
29. Thomas Raynalde and Eucharius Rösslin, *The Byrth of Mankynde, Otherwyse Named the Womans Booke* (London: By Thomas Raynalde, 1545). Elizabeth Lane Furdell, *Publishing and Medicine in Early Modern England* (Rochester, NY: University of Rochester Press, 2002), pp. 29–48.
30. Alessandro Massaria and Robert Turner, *De Morbis Foemineis, the Womans Counsellour: Or, the Feminine Physitian* (London: Printed for John Streater, 1657). François Mauriceau, *The Diseases of Women with Child and in Child-Bed* (London: Printed by John Darby, 1683).

31. Nicholas Culpeper, *A Directory for Midwives: Or, a Guide for Women, in Their Conception, Bearing, and Suckling Their Children* (London: Printed by Peter Cole, 1651). Jane Sharp, *The Midwives Book, or, the Whole Art of Midwifry Discovered* (London: Printed for Simon Miller 1671).
32. *The English Midwife Enlarged* (London: Printed for Thomas Sawbridge 1682).
33. Mary Rhinelander McCarl, 'Publishing the Works of Nicholas Culpeper, Astrological Herbalist and Translator of Latin Medical Works in Seventeenth-Century London', *Canadian Bulletin of Medical History* 13, no. 2 (1996): 225–276.
34. Mary Fissell, 'Hairy Women and Naked Truths: Gender and the Politics of Knowledge in "Aristotle's Masterpiece"', *William and Mary Quarterly* (2003): 43–75. Vern L Bullough, 'An Early American Sex Manual, or, Aristotle Who?,' *Early American Literature* 7, no. 3 (1973): 236–246. Fissell, 'Making a Masterpiece: The Aristotle Texts in Vernacular Medical Culture'.
35. Fissell, *Vernacular Bodies*, p. 2.
36. Wear, *Knowledge and Practice in English Medicine*, pp. 40–50. Alexandra Halasz, *The Marketplace of Print: Pamphlets and the Public Sphere in Early Modern England* (Cambridge: Cambridge University Press, 2006), p. 56.
37. Culpeper, *A Directory for Midwives.* Sharp, *The Midwives Book.* James Wolveridge, *Speculum Matricis Hybernicum, or, the Irish Midwives Handmaid* (London: Printed by E. Okes, 1670).
38. Nicholas Sudell, *Mulierum Amicus: Or, the Womans Friend* (London: 1666). Robert Barret, *A Companion for Midwives, Child-Bearing Women, and Nurses Directing Them How to Perform Their Respective Offices* (London: Printed for Thomas Ax, 1699).
39. Culpeper, *A Directory for Midwives*, epistle dedicatory.
40. Sudell, *Mulierum Amicus: Or, the Womans Friend*, A3. See also: Daphna Oren-Magidor, 'Literate Laywomen, Male Medical Practitioners and the Treatment of Fertility Problems in Early Modern England', *Social History of Medicine* 29, no. 2 (2016): 290–310.
41. Jennifer Evans, '"The Doctor's Wife (by the Blessing of God) Helps Barrenness": Gender and Infertility Treatments in Early Modern England', in *Gender, Health and Medicine in Historical Perspective (Provisional Title)*, ed. Sarah Toulalan, p. 14. My thanks to Jennifer Evans for advance access to this paper. Dorothy Porter and Roy Porter, *Patient's Progress: Doctors and Doctoring in Eighteenth-Century England* (Stanford, CA: Stanford University Press, 1989), p. 204. Mary Glover, *Medical Recipes*, BL Add. MSS 57944, f. 10v. Elaine Leong, '"Herbals She Peruseth": Reading Medicine in Early Modern England', *Renaissance Studies* 28, no. 4 (2014): 556–578.

42. Porter and Porter, *Patient's Progress: Doctors and Doctoring in Eighteenth-Century England*, p. 204. Fissell, 'Making a Masterpiece: The Aristotle Texts in Vernacular Medical Culture', p. 204. Jennifer Evans, *Aphrodisiacs, Fertility and Medicine in Early Modern England* (London: Royal Historical Society, 2014), pp. 34–36.
43. A. Marsh, *The Ten Pleasures of Marriage Relating All the Delights and Contentments That Are Mask'd under the Bands of Matrimony* (London: 1682), p. 79.
44. Bridget MacCarthy, *The Female Pen: Women Writers and Novelists, 1621–1818* (New York: NYU Press, 1946), pp. 169–240. The preface to this edition, page xix, points out that MacCarthy's attempt to attribute this text to Aphra Behn has generally been rejected by newer literary scholarship, but that her analysis more broadly is still sound.
45. McLaren, *Reproductive Rituals*, pp. 16–17.
46. Massaria and Turner, *De Morbis Foemineis*, pp. 94–95.
47. Massaria and Turner, *De Morbis Foemineis*, p. 95.
48. Culpeper, *A Directory for Midwives*, pp. 83–114.
49. Nicholas Culpeper, *Directory for Midwives* (London, 1671), p. 135.
50. Jakob Rueff, 'Book 6,' in *The Expert Midwife, or an Excellent and Most Necessary Treatise of the Generation and Birth of Man* (London: Printed by E. Griffin for S. Burton, 1637), p. 13.
51. Alan Macfarlane, *Marriage and Love in England: Modes of Reproduction 1300–1840* (Oxford: Blackwell, 1986), p. 61.
52. Massaria and Turner, *De Morbis Foemineis*, p. 103.
53. Massaria and Turner, *De Morbis Foemineis*, p. 103.
54. Nicolaas Fonteyn, *The Womans Doctour, or, an Exact and Distinct Explanation of All Such Diseases as Are Peculiar to That Sex* (London: Printed for John Blague and Samuel Howes, 1652), pp. 128–129.
55. *The Compleat Midwifes Practice, in the Most Weighty and High Concernments of the Birth of Man Containing Perfect Rules for Midwifes and Nurses* (London: Printed for Nathaniel Brooke, 1656), pp. 66–67.
56. Mauriceau, *The Diseases of Women with Child and in Child-Bed*, p. 7.
57. Fonteyn, *The Womans Doctour*, pp. 129–130.
58. Fonteyn, *The Womans Doctour*, pp. 129–130.
59. *Aristoteles Master-Piece, or, the Secrets of Generation Displayed in All the Parts Thereof* (London: Printed for J. How, 1684), pp. 58–59.
60. *The Compleat Midwifes Practice*, p. 68.
61. Massaria and Turner, *De Morbis Foemineis*, pp. 116–117.
62. Fissell, 'Gender and Generation: Representing Reproduction in Early Modern England', 440. On agricultural metaphors see also: Smith, 'Imagining Women's Fertility Before Technology', 70.
63. Sharp, *The Midwives Book*, p. 92.

64. Culpeper, *A Directory for Midwives*, p. 135.
65. Smith, 'Imagining Women's Fertility Before Technology', 72.
66. Cathy McClive, 'Menstrual Knowledge and Medical Practice in Early Modern France, c. 1555–1761', in *Menstruation: A Cultural History*, ed. Andrew Shail and Gillian Howie (Basingstoke: Palgrave Macmillan, 2005). Patricia Crawford, 'Attitudes to Menstruation in Seventeenth-Century England', *Past & Present*, no. 91 (1981): 47–73.
67. Culpeper, *A Directory for Midwives*, p. 86.
68. *The Compleat Midwifes Practice*, p. 70.
69. Massaria and Turner, *De Morbis Foemineis*, p. 118.
70. Rueff, 'Book 6', p. 13.
71. Rueff, 'Book 6', p. 13.
72. Jennifer Evans, '"They Are Called Imperfect Men": Male Infertility and Sexual Health in Early Modern England', *Social History of Medicine* 29, no. 2 (2014): 311–332.
73. Massaria and Turner, *De Morbis Foemineis*, p. 105.
74. The question of whether a man with damaged genitalia could marry was not entirely straightforward, as is evidenced by Helen Berry's detailed exploration of the marriage and subsequent trial of the castrato Giusto Fernando Tenducci in the eighteenth century. Helen Berry, *The Castrato and His Wife* (Oxford: Oxford University Press, 2011).
75. Massaria and Turner, *De Morbis Foemineis*, p. 107.
76. Sharp, *The Midwives Book*, 83. Helkiah Crooke, *Mikrokosmographia a Description of the Body of Man.* (London: Printed by William Iaggard, 1615), p. 219.
77. Massaria and Turner, *De Morbis Foemineis*, p. 109.
78. On male infertility see Evans, '"They Are Called Imperfect Men": Male Infertility and Sexual Health in Early Modern England'. Catherine Rider, 'Men and Infertility in Late Medieval English Medicine', *Social History of Medicine* 29, no. 2 (2016): 245–266. Helen Berry and Elizabeth A. Foyster, 'Childless Men in Early Modern England', in *The Family in Early Modern England*, ed. Helen Berry and Elizabeth A. Foyster (Cambridge: Cambridge University Press, 2007).
79. Gowing, *Gender Relations in Early Modern England*, p. 8.
80. Fonteyn, *The Womans Doctour*, p. 133. Incontinent here in the sense of lacking restraint.
81. Merry E. Wiesner, *Women and Gender in Early Modern Europe* (Cambridge: Cambridge University Press, 2000), p. 19. Bernard Capp, *When Gossips Meet: Women, Family, and Neighbourhood in Early Modern England* (Oxford: Oxford University Press, 2003), p. 12. Mark Breitenberg, *Anxious Masculinity in Early Modern England* (Cambridge: Cambridge University Press, 1996), pp. 20, 48.

82. '"Frigid, Adj."', in *Oxford English Dictionary* (Oxford University Press).
83. Rueff, 'Book 6', p. 14. Wiesner, *Women and Gender in Early Modern Europe*, p. 18.
84. Rueff, 'Book 6', p. 14.
85. Rueff, 'Book 6', p. 14.
86. Massaria and Turner, *De Morbis Foemineis*, p. 119.
87. *Aristoteles Master-Piece*, p. 60.
88. Foyster, *Manhood in Early Modern England*, pp. 9–10.
89. Harvey, 'The History of Masculinity, Circa 1650–1800', 298.
90. Fonteyn, *The Womans Doctour*, pp. 131–132.
91. Massaria and Turner, *De Morbis Foemineis*, pp. 111–112.
92. Massaria and Turner, *De Morbis Foemineis*, p. 111. *The English Midwife Enlarged*, p. 189.
93. Sarah Toulalan, '"To[O] Much Eating Stifles the Child": Fat Bodies and Reproduction in Early Modern England', *Historical Research* 87, no. 235 (2014): 65–93.
94. Massaria and Turner, *De Morbis Foemineis*, pp. 111–112.
95. Wolveridge, *Speculum Matricis Hybernicum, or, the Irish Midwives Handmaid*, pp. 106–107.
96. Culpeper, *A Directory for Midwives*, p. 115.
97. Wolveridge, *Speculum Matricis Hybernicum, or, the Irish Midwives Handmaid*, pp. 106–107. *The Compleat Midvvife's Practice Enlarged* (London: Printed for Nathaniel Brooke, 1659), p. 68.
98. Sharp, *The Midwives Book*, p. 90.
99. Massaria and Turner, *De Morbis Foemineis*, pp. 118–119. Wolveridge, *Speculum Matricis Hybernicum, or, the Irish Midwives Handmaid*, pp. 106–107.
100. W.A. Speck, 'Mary II (1662–1694)', in *Oxford Dictionary of National Biography, Online ed.*, ed. Lawrence Goldman (Oxford: Oxford University Press, 2004). Mary Anne Everett Green, *Letters of Queen Henrietta Maria, Including Her Private Correspondence with Charles I* (London: Richard Bentley), pp. 14–15.
101. Gail Kern Paster, *The Body Embarrassed: Drama and the Disciplines of Shame in Early Modern England* (Ithaca, NY: Cornell University Press, 1993), p. 181.
102. Paster, *The Body Embarrassed*, p. 181.
103. *The Compleat Midvvife's Practice Enlarged*, p. 67. Wolveridge, *Speculum Matricis Hybernicum, or, the Irish Midwives Handmaid*, pp. 106–107.
104. Gwynne Kennedy, *Just Anger: Representing Women's Anger in Early Modern England* (Bloomington: South Indiana University Press, 2000), p. 19.
105. Foyster, *Manhood in Early Modern England*, p. 188.

106. Ulinka Rublack, 'Pregnancy, Childbirth and the Female Body in Early Modern Germany', *Past & Present*, no. 150 (1996): 84–110.
107. Adrian Wilson, *Ritual and Conflict: The Social Relations of Childbirth in Early Modern England* (England: Ashgate, 2016), p. 98.
108. William Gouge, *Of Domesticall Duties* (London: Printed by Iohn Haviland for William Bladen, 1622), pp. 221–222. See also: Thomas A. Foster, 'Deficient Husbands: Manhood, Sexual Incapacity, and Male Marital Sexuality in Seventeenth-Century New England', *The William and Mary Quarterly* 56, no. 4 (1999): 723–744. Frye Roland Mushat, 'The Teachings of Classical Puritanism on Conjugal Love', *Studies in the Renaissance* 2 (1955): 148–159.
109. Gouge, *Of Domesticall Duties*, p. 225.
110. Wilson, *Ritual and Conflict*, pp. 88–92.
111. On the ideals of marriage, especially affectionate marriage, see Diana O'Hara, *Courtship and Constraint: Rethinking the Making of Marriage in Tudor England* (Manchester: Manchester University Press, 2000). Lawrence Stone, *The Family, Sex and Marriage in England, 1500–1800* (New York: Harper & Row, 1977). Robert Brink Shoemaker, *Gender in English Society, 1650–1850: The Emergence of Separate Spheres?* (London: Longman, 1998), p. 90. Macfarlane, *Marriage and Love in England.*
112. Thomas Walter Laqueur, *Making Sex: Body and Gender from the Greeks to Freud* (Cambridge, MA: Harvard University Press, 1990), pp. 1–2. Shoemaker, *Gender in English Society, 1650–1850*, pp. 60–62. McLaren, *Reproductive Rituals*, p. 20.
113. Lazare Rivière, *The Practice of Physick in Seventeen Several Books* (London: Printed by Peter Cole, 1655), p. 503.
114. *The Compleat Midvvife's Practice Enlarged*, pp. 44, 67–68.
115. *The English Midwife Enlarged*, pp. 177–178.
116. Fonteyn, *The Womans Doctour*, pp. 133–135.
117. *The English Midwife Enlarged*, p. 191.
118. Mauriceau, *The Diseases of Women with Child and in Child-Bed*, p. 7. *The English Midwife Enlarged*, p. 191.
119. Jacques Guillemeau, *Child-Birth or, the Happy Deliuerie of Vvomen* (London: Printed by A. Hatfield, 1612), p. 3.
120. Evans, *Aphrodisiacs, Fertility and Medicine in Early Modern England.*
121. Foster, 'Deficient Husbands: Manhood, Sexual Incapacity, and Male Marital Sexuality in Seventeenth-Century New England'. Roland Mushat, 'The Teachings of Classical Puritanism on Conjugal Love'. Wiesner, *Women and Gender in Early Modern Europe.*
122. Sharp, *The Midwives Book*, pp. 99–100.
123. *Aristoteles Master-Piece*, p. 59.
124. O'Hara, *Courtship and Constraint.*

125. Christine Peters, 'Gender, Sacrament and Ritual: The Making and Meaning of Marriage in Late Medieval and Early Modern England', *Past & Present*, no. 169 (2000): 63–96.
126. Culpeper, *A Directory for Midwives*, pp. 85–86.
127. Philip Barrough, *The Methode of Phisicke Conteyning the Causes, Signes, and Cures of Invvard Diseases in Mans Body* (Imprinted at London: By Thomas Vautroullier, 1583), p. 157.
128. Culpeper, *Directory for Midwives*, p. 133. McLaren, *Reproductive Rituals*, pp. 21–22.
129. Michal Altbauer-Rudnik, 'Love Madness and Social Order: Love Melancholy in France and England in the Late Sixteenth and Early Seventeenth Centuries', *Gesnerus* 63, no. 1/2 (2006): 33–45.
130. Culpeper, *A Directory for Midwives*, pp. 84–85. Sharp, *The Midwives Book*, pp. 99–100.
131. Sara Heller Mendelson and Mary O'Connor, '"Thy Passionately Loving Sister and Faithfull Friend": Anne Dormer's Letters to Her Sister Lady Trumbull', in *Sibling Relations and Gender in the Early Modern World: Sisters, Brothers and Others*, ed. Naomi J. Miller and Naomi Yavneh (Aldershot: Ashgate, 2006).
132. Alan Macfarlane, 'Illegitimacy and Illegitimates in English History', in *Bastardy and Its Comparative History: Studies in the History of Illegitimacy and Marital Nonconformism in Britain, France, Germany, Sweden, North America, Jamaica, and Japan*, ed. Peter Laslett, Karla Oosterveen and Richard Michael Smith (Cambridge, MA: Harvard University Press, 1980).
133. *Aristoteles Master-Piece*, p. 59. Sharp, *The Midwives Book*, pp. 99–100.
134. Laura Gowing, *Common Bodies: Women, Touch and Power in Seventeenth-Century England* (New Haven, CT: Yale University Press, 2003), p. 91.
135. Maclean, 'Evidence, Logic, the Rule and the Exception in Renaissance Law and Medicine', 232.
136. Lorraine Daston, 'Marvelous Facts and Miraculous Evidence in Early Modern Europe', *Critical Inquiry* 18, no. 1 (1991): 112.
137. Daston, 'Marvelous Facts and Miraculous Evidence in Early Modern Europe', 248.
138. Walsham, *Providence in Early Modern England*, pp. 27–28.
139. Lauren Kassell, *Medicine and Magic in Elizabethan London: Simon Forman: Astrologer, Alchemist, and Physician* (Oxford: Oxford University Press, 2007), pp. 9–12.
140. William Drage, *Daimonomageia: A Small Treatise of Sicknesses and Diseases from Witchcraft, and Supernatural Causes* (London: Printed by J. Dover, 1665), p. 10.
141. Fonteyn, *The Womans Doctour*, pp. 136–137.
142. Culpeper, *A Directory for Midwives*, pp. 112–113.

143. Rueff, 'Book 6', 16. *The Compleat Midwifes Practice*, p. 67. Sudell, *Mulierum Amicus: Or, the Womans Friend*, 49. Sharp, *The Midwives Book*, p. 101.
144. Sharp, *The Midwives Book*, p. 101.
145. Jacques Gélis, *History of Childbirth: Fertility, Pregnancy and Birth in Early Modern Europe* (Boston, MA: Rosemary Morris, 1991), pp. 26–27.
146. Owen Davies, *Popular Magic: Cunning Folk in English History* (London: Hambledon Continuum, 2007).
147. James Sharpe, *English Witchcraft, 1560–1736*, (London: Pickering & Chatto, 2003), pp. 296, 317.
148. Sharpe, *English Witchcraft, 1560–1736*, pp. 296, 317.
149. *Damnable Practises of Three Lincolne-Shire Witches, Joane Flower, and Her Two Daughters, Margret and Phillip Flower* (London: Printed by G. Eld for Iohn Barnes, 1619).
150. Lyndal Roper, *Oedipus and the Devil: Witchcraft, Sexuality, and Religion in Early Modern Europe* (London; New York: Routledge, 1994), pp. 200–210.
151. Cecil Henry L'Estrange Ewen, *Witchcraft and Demonianism: A Concise Account Derived from Sworn Depositions and Confessions Obtained in the Courts of England and Wale* (London: Muller, 1970), p. 317.
152. Ewen, *Witchcraft and Demonianism*, p. 246.
153. James Sharpe, *Witchcraft in Early Modern England* (Harlow, England Longman, 2001), pp. 13, 24. Brian P. Levack, *The Witch-Hunt in Early Modern Europe* (London Longman, 1989), pp. 67–69.
154. Culpeper, *A Directory for Midwives*, pp. 112–113.
155. *Book of Magical Charms*, BL Sloane MS 1311, f. 89.
156. Lyndal Roper, *Witch Craze: Terror and Fantasy in Baroque Germany* (New Haven, CT: Yale University Press, 2004), p. 32.
157. Gélis, *History of Childbirth*, pp. 15, 26–27.
158. Bernard Cottret, *The Huguenots in England: Immigration and Settlement, c. 1550–1700* (Cambridge: Cambridge University Press, 1991). Nigel Goose and Liên Luu, *Immigrants in Tudor and Early Stuart England* (Brighton: Sussex Academic Press, 2005).
159. Sarah Toulalan, *Imagining Sex: Pornography and Bodies in Seventeenth-Century England* (Oxford: Oxford University Press, 2007), pp. 18, 65. Anna Bayman, '"Large Hands, Wide Eares, and Piercing Sights": The "Discoveries" of the Elizabethan and Jacobean Witch Pamphlets', *Literature & History* 16, no. 1 (2007): 26–45.

CHAPTER 4

Society and Infertility

In June 1677 a strange infanticide case came before the Old Bailey, involving a midwife from St Giles Cripplegate parish in London.[1] The story was unusual enough that it was retold as a ballad, printed sometime before 1679.[2] The ballad and the Old Bailey proceedings differ on the details of the case but the basic story remains consistent in both of them. It is the story of a midwife who had been married for some time, perhaps even several times, but did not conceive. She decided to fake a pregnancy by hiding a pillow under her clothes to simulate a growing belly, and when it was time for her to go into labour she used her professional connections to procure a dead infant, then pretended to give birth to a stillborn child. The midwife was accused of deliberately killing a child in order to present it as her own and was arrested for infanticide. Upon hearing witness testimony, however, the court ruled that while the midwife's actions were motivated by a 'strange extravagant humour', she had not killed a child, and she was therefore set free.[3]

The story itself is interesting enough, but it is the reasoning offered for actions that is particularly significant, as it highlights the social pressures placed on infertile women. The ballad explained that the midwife wanted to prove to her neighbours 'That she from Barrenness was free, and fruitful as the best'.[4] The court records claimed that she had faked the pregnancy because she wanted to 'satisfie her husband, who was very impatient to have a child' and 'to preserve her credit in her imploy

D. Oren-Magidor, *Infertility in Early Modern England*,
Early Modern History: Society and Culture,
DOI 10.1057/978-1-137-47668-5_4

which she thought somewhat prejudiced by the imputation of barrenness'.[5] These two explanations demonstrate that a woman's fertility, or lack thereof, was not only a matter for her husband, her family or her closest friends. It was something that her neighbours discussed and that affected her personal and professional reputation. The majority of London midwives in this period did have children of their own, and often completed their childbearing cycle before licensing, so that a childless midwife was quite uncommon.[6] It is worthy of note that if the court records are correct about her motives, the midwife of St Giles believed that giving birth to a stillborn child would improve her reputation, so that even an unsuccessful pregnancy was better than none. Perhaps people expected a midwife to have some personal experience with childbirth even if it did not result in a living child. In any case, infertility caused sufficient damage to a woman's reputation that it was seen as plausible, albeit strange, that she would go to the trouble of faking a stillbirth simply to avoid the 'imputation of barrenness'.[7] The midwife's actions were seen as an extreme response to infertility, an 'extravagant humour', but they were not understood as completely senseless. Indeed, in a society that placed considerable pressure on married couples to have children, the midwife's actions can be seen as an attempt to curb the social consequences of a medical condition she could not cure.

It is difficult to trace the actual social impact of being infertile. There is only very limited evidence of specific individuals being mocked because they were childless, and it is not the aim of this chapter to claim that all or even most childless couples in England were subject to public ridicule and derision. Rather, it is to say that early modern English culture contained a recurring and prominent negative attitude toward infertile people, both men and women. This was not the only way that early modern people understood and addressed infertility, but it made up a significant portion of the cultural and social discussions of fertility problems in this period. A satirical piece on marriage dating from 1621 described the private and public shame that men endured when their wives were barren and the inherently emasculating nature of this shame: 'if [the wife] is barren, the husband lives then in great discontent, esteeming himself to be in hatred with God and nature, in being denied that comfort, for which chiefly he married: And not giving him the fruite of that blessing, the want whereof maketh him reproachfull, whereby he shameth to accompany with men, as seeing himself to be lesse then [*sic*] a man'.[8] It is significant that there is no separation here between the man and his wife in terms of the consequences of infertility. The wife is 'barren', but the reproach falls on both the wife and her husband.

The negative attitude towards infertile people appeared in multiple contexts, including medical writing, religious guidebooks, 'popular' and 'high' literature, political polemic and more. Examined together, these views contain several key elements:

1) That infertility might be a punishment for sins, and therefore that infertile people were, potentially, sinners.
2) That infertile women tended, by their nature, to be lustful and promiscuous.
3) That infertile women tended to be outspoken and domineering, and therefore transgressing of the expected behaviour for 'proper' women. Conversely, women who were notorious for transgressing gender boundaries by speaking out where they should not or behaving in an 'unwomanly' fashion were described as suffering from reproductive failures, usually miscarriages or even monstrous births.
4) That infertile men were effeminate and weak and that they were unable to exercise self-control and, more importantly, to control their wives.

While there were some expressions of negative views of infertility that contained only some of these elements, the significance of the combination between the four becomes clear in the recurrence—again, in several different cultural spheres—of one particular trope: the barren woman who becomes 'cured' of her infertility and successfully bears a child after she commits adultery. The 'adulterous barren woman' story contains within it the promiscuous and lustful barren woman, who also transgresses the boundaries of proper womanly behaviour, and the weak and ineffectual husband—implicitly the true source of the couple's infertility—who cannot control his wife sufficiently to keep her faithful. The prevalent view of infertility thus connects directly with the 'contested' status of gender relations in early modern England, identified by Adrian Wilson. Wilson argues that in early modern culture 'Alongside the figures of the dutiful wife and ruling husband stood their equally familiar transgressive counter parts, the "shrew" and the "skimmington:" that is, the wife who "wore the breeches" and the husband who let her do so.'[9] Wilson identifies this contested status as related to the economic sphere, noting that often self-assertive women in England were also those of greater economic independence.[10] Mark Breitenberg also argues that early modern gender relations were in a state of constant 'anxiety', stating that masculinity is inherently anxious in a patriarchal system, because 'individuals whose identities are formed by the assumption of their own privilege must also have incorporated varying degrees of anxiety about the preservation or potential loss of that privilege'.[11] The trope of the adulterous barren woman ties together these different forms of anxiety, and gives them an expression that is not directly related to economic relations, nor is it about marital authority per se. Instead, it highlights a fear that the sexual, dominating and transgressive wife would perform the ultimate trick on her weak and ineffectual husband. She would be 'cured' of her own problematic infertility, while not only cuckolding her husband but also presenting another man's child as his own. Whatever mockery infertile individuals did or did not face, then, infertility in itself was understood as unsettling to the social order. Indeed, as Lisa Smith argues, 'Sterility was potentially as destabilizing to a community as concealed pregnancies.'[12]

Barren Sinners

Women were long understood to have a strong potential for sin, and this sin was often punished through women's bodies and in particular through their reproductive faculties.[13] Eve, the ultimate sinner, was punished for her sin by being made to suffer through childbirth, and this was extended to all women, as John Oliver wrote in 1663: 'sin makes travel [labour] painful'.[14] Martin Luther stated that 'although women had brought about the Fall, they were sanctified by the bearing of children', and English preachers followed suit, linking fertility with salvation. But if women were saved through childbearing, then it might follow that a woman who did not bear children was not saved.[15] At best, religious authors presented infertility as a difficult test to be endured. At worst, it was 'a just punishment for an incontinent life', as Abraham Wright put it in his commentary on the book of Genesis.[16]

In medical texts, the implied connection between infertility and sin was described as a reason to treat it promptly, to assist women in avoiding the stigmas associated with childlessness. *The English Midwife* (1682) stated in its section on barrenness that in Biblical times 'some like *Rachel* have cry'd out to their Husbands for children . . . rather than endure the reproach of barrenness'. It continued to argue that 'you shall find but few Women of their minds now a days'.[17] Alan Macfarlane uses this statement in order to argue that infertility was not seen as a form of divine punishment in early modern England. But the text, copied almost verbatim from the translation of Alessandro Massaria's midwifery manual of 1657, was by no means typical.[18] In 1656 Richard Bunworth published *The Doctresse*, a book of cures for women's illnesses. Bunworth described the effects of one remedy for barrenness by stating that 'this, by God's blessing, will make her that is barren a happy mother, and take away her reproach amongst women'.[19] Robert Johnson's 1683 medical manual similarly showed a similar awareness of the distress that infertility caused women. He wrote that 'very few Women in a Marriage state but desire Children, yea some would give all they have in the world for a Child, and are very impatient if they do not Conceive. *Rachel* said to *Jacob* in *Gen.* 30 ver. I. *Give me Children, or else I dye.*'[20] Johnson saw the Biblical references as relevant to his reader's own lives, as indeed they were.[21] When he wrote 'We reade in the Scripture, that the Women of old did think it a reproach to be Childless', he was not claiming that things were different in his own times, but that this was relevant to his readers, and that infertility ought to be cured in order to prevent such reproach.[22]

There is more direct evidence that women in seventeenth-century England also viewed infertility as a 'reproach'. Laura Gowing's study of defamation cases in London suggests that fertility was used as proof of a woman's morality and infertility as a sign of immorality. Gowing notes the case of two London women in the seventeenth century in which one told the other that 'I have ten children, and thou has never a one', and that of a woman who responded to being called a bitch by saying 'I have been the mother of sixteen children', as though the very fact of having children automatically negated the insult. In yet another case one woman brought a defamation case against another for saying that she would never have children, because this implied that she was promiscuous.[23] Evidence from other locations in England indicates that the birth of a stillborn or deformed child might also be interpreted as punishment for sexual or religious immorality.[24]

The idea that infertility was a marker of immorality had some cultural power. It appeared, for example, in ballads, a popular literary form that circulated in both literate and illiterate crowds, and is therefore a useful marker for identifying cultural attitudes that were familiar to various parts of English society.[25] Nicholas Bownde wrote in 1595 that in the shops and homes of artisans and poorer husbandmen 'you shall sooner see one of these new ballads than any of the psalms', and ballads were sung in markets and village commons, making them accessible to a wide audience.[26] Ballads were a literary device meant both to entertain their readers and listeners and to disseminate ideas about morality, religion or appropriate behaviour. Because they aimed at entertainment and titillation, ballads often told exaggerated or fabulous stories, but this did not mean that they did not reflect certain social values, expressed both implicitly and explicitly in the ballads' stories. *The Old Man's Complaint*, a ballad published in about 1629, told a story that tied greed and mistreatment of an elderly parent with childlessness and its attendant social stigma. The ballad told the story of an old man whose son and daughter-in-law, a wealthy couple, did not treat him well. Despite their wealth and their comfortable living, the son and his wife were miserable, because they had no children. The wife, in particular, was willing to do anything to have a child, not least because of the social reproach associated with childlessness:

> Quote she a hundred pound would I give for a child:
> To have a jolly child:
> Of mine owne body borne;
> Full oft I am revil'd,
> Of this my barren wombe.[27]

Within a few years the son died of his misery, and the old man inherited his fortune and lived out the rest of his life in comfort and joy. Whatever joys the couple may have had were utterly destroyed by their inability to bear children (a plot device which enabled the old man to inherit at their deaths). The ballad described infertility not only as an emotional difficulty, but also as a social hardship, because the wife did not only desire children for their own sake but also because she was 'revil'd' for her barrenness. It also, however, made a clear connection between the abuse of the father and the suffering of the son. Childlessness and its miseries were presented as a just punishment for a son who did not respect his father.

Women could also use barrenness as an actual curse, wishing infertility upon their enemies. When the target of Anne Murray's (later Anne, Lady Halkett) affections married another woman, Murray's maid Miriam acted in anger and 'shee lifted up her hands and said, 'Give her [the wife], O Lord, dry breasts and a miscarying wombe, a curse which 'the Lord thought fitt to grant'.[28] The fact that the maid chose to curse the couple with childlessness is indicative both of the importance of reproduction in this society and of the degree to which infertility was perceived as a stain. It is also telling that while it was the man who had wronged her mistress, Miriam chose to curse his wife rather than him directly. By cursing the wife to childlessness, Miriam was taking her revenge on both members of the couple. A husband could be punished through his wife's body and the loss of her reproductive abilities, suggesting that a woman's reproduction was almost an extension of her husband, something belonging to him which could be taken away in order to punish him for his actions. Clergyman Donald Lupton claimed in 1634 that God threatened to give '*dry* breasts, and *barren* wombs as a curse to *sinfull*, and *disobedient* Husbands'.[29] The wife's womb and her breasts belonged to her husband, and were therefore available to be used as punishment.

Quotidian infertility might be seen as a sign of immorality, but there was a more powerful articulation of the connection between sin, reproductive failure and the transgression of gendered boundaries. This came in the form of fantastical tales of 'monstrous births', which were not only events of failed reproduction, but events in which childbearing was unnatural and subverted. These were used to criticize, marginalize and ostracize women who were seen as threatening to the very social order. Julie Crawford argues that monstrous births 'do not just appear; they are made, and understood to be made, in women's bodies. It is *women* whose acts and behaviours produce monsters.'[30] Moreover, David Cressy claims that stories of monstrous birth and other reproductive oddities emerged 'from the contested culture of post-Reformation England', and that such stories were 'rooted in local struggles and shaped by contests over gender, authority, deference and belief'.[31] Stories of monstrous births sometimes had a grain of truth in that they were based on cases of miscarriage or stillbirth, but these relatively commonplace occurrences were elaborated and expanded to create an image of a woman so sinful and so dangerous to the natural order that her very body rejected its proper feminine role and produced misshapen children.

One such fantastical story appeared in the legend of the Countess Margaret of Henneberg, who was punished for sinful behaviour by giving birth to 365 stillborn babies (or short-lived babies, depending on the version of the story). The legend itself originated in the Netherlands in the thirteenth century and a monument commemorating the titillating birth can still be seen in the church at Loosduinen, which was even believed to have magical abilities to restore fertility.[32] The legend gained a great deal of popularity in England in the sixteenth and seventeenth centuries. Hyder E. Rollins surveys the mentions of this legend in Europe in this period, most of them from England, and finds it occurring approximately forty times.[33] Even Rollin's survey is not comprehensive. He notes that Samuel Pepys went to visit the memorial at Loosduineen, but does not mention that Jane Sharp referred to the story in her *Midwife's Book*, albeit describing it as 'Meer Romance'.[34] The version of the legend that likely received the widest circulation and would have been the most approachable to an illiterate as well as a literate audience, appeared in a ballad printed in about 1620, entitled *The Lamenting Lady*.[35] The ballad did not mention Henneberg by name, nor did the story take place in any specific location, but the story is clearly the same. The ballad told of a rich lady who lamented that she had no children and felt this was particularly unfair because she was so wealthy and lived such a cultured and gentle life, while many beggars and poor women had children. No explicit connection was made between the lady's behaviour and her barrenness, but it was implied that her rich lifestyle and disdain of poor people contributed to her state. The lady's punishment, in the form of reproductive misery, came as a result of her directly mistreating another person, a beggar woman with two children who appeared at her door. The lady swore at the beggar and told her that her children must be the result of infidelity, because otherwise a beggar woman should not have children when a rich lady had none. The beggar woman responded by cursing the lady, telling her that she would give birth, at one time, to as many children as there were days in the year. The beggar's curse came true and the lady suffered through an unnatural pregnancy that robbed her of her beauty, finally giving birth to hundreds of stillborn children, all of whom were buried together.

Ballads were not only a verbal medium, meant to be read or sung. They were also a visual medium in which the images conveyed messages to illiterate or partially literate audiences.[36] The print edition of the ballad *The Lamenting Lady* contained two images that illustrated the moral that the mistreatment of the beggar woman by the rich lady led to the lady's reproductive suffering. The Fig. 4.1 shows the lady, richly dressed, berating the poor woman (recognized by her simpler garb) who is holding two small babies. In Fig. 4.2 the lady is lying in her bed praying, while her husband also demonstrates his woe, while on the table near them lies a casket full of perfectly formed but stillborn babies. Although the images do not tell the whole story of the ballad, they illustrate the sin (turning away the beggar woman) and its consequences (the dead children).

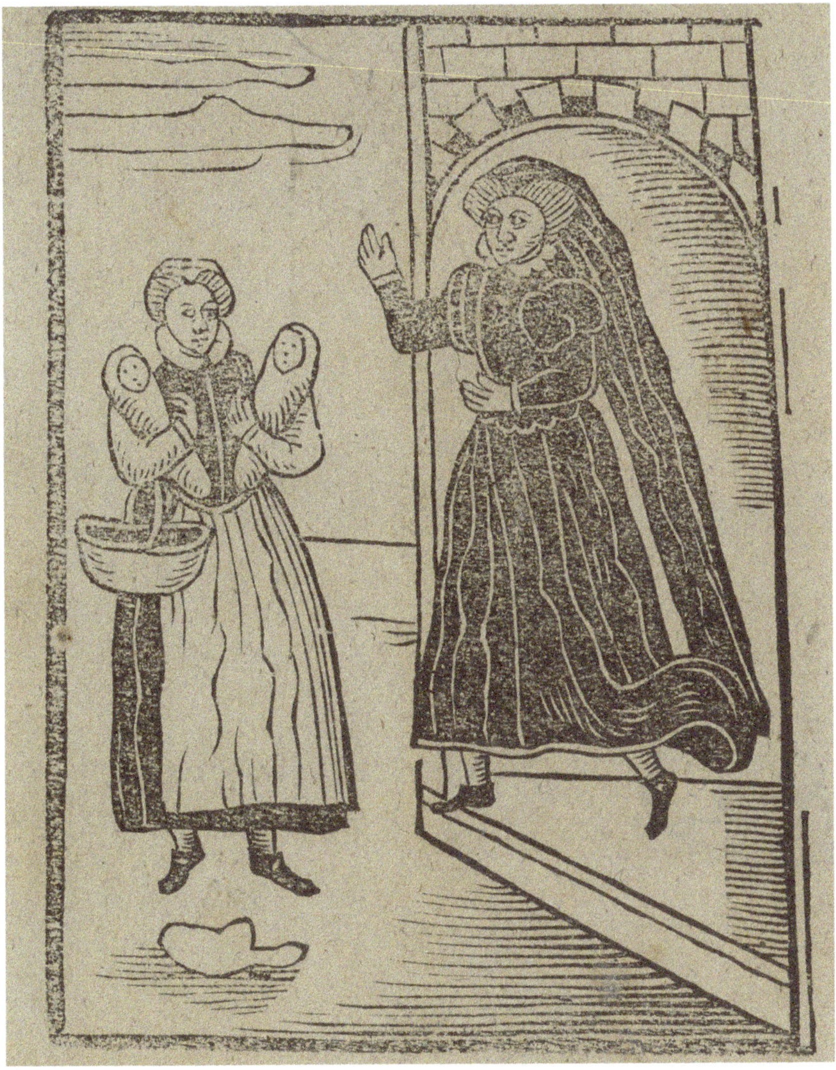

Fig. 4.1 The Lady turns away a beggar woman, by permission of the Pepys Library, Magdalene College, Cambridge

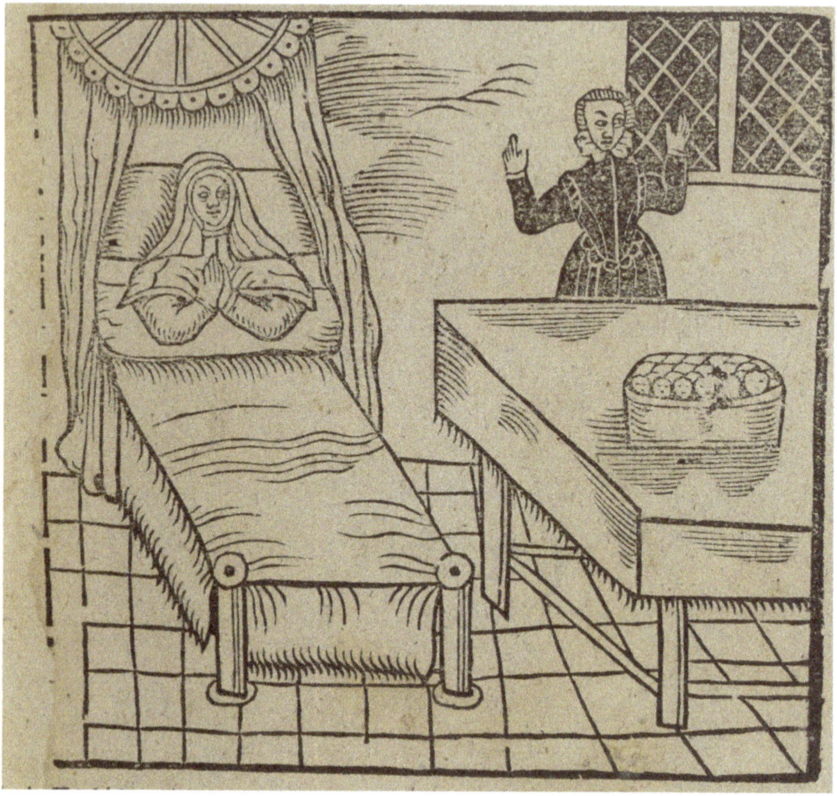

Fig. 4.2 The Lady and her 365 babies, by permission of the Pepys Library, Magdalene College, Cambridge

The story of the 365 babies was meant as a moral tale, an obvious legend with a good lesson at its side. Monstrous births, however, were not relegated only to the realm of the fantastical, but were used in real cases in order to criticize and even ostracize real women. Nowhere is this more evident than in the trials of Anne Hutchinson and her followers in Massachusetts in the 1630s, in which reproductive tragedy was used in order to attempt to put women back in their 'proper' place. There are some obvious differences between the society of the New England colonies and English society, but in the 1630s most of the residents of New England were born and educated in England and the majority of their cultural values and ideas came from England, specifically from the 'godly' or 'Puritan' subculture. Because migrants to New England typically arrived as families, rather than single men looking for work, the composition of New England society more closely replicated English society than other immigrant communities in the British colonies.[37] Therefore, evidence from the early days of English settlement in New England can be revealing of cultural beliefs in England itself.

Hutchinson first gained attention by hosting Bible meetings which went against the teachings of the organized Church in Massachusetts. These meetings were initially attended only by women, but later began attracting men as well. Hutchinson and her followers were tried for blasphemy and accused of being heretics as well as for sexual depravity, and the colony's leaders ultimately excommunicated them and banished them to what would become the colony of Rhode Island. John Winthrop, governor and one of the founders of the Massachusetts Bay Colony as well as a staunch Puritan, took great pains to discredit Hutchinson and her followers in the strictest possible terms.[38] Winthrop's propaganda included a description of several cases of monstrous birth which had supposedly occurred within Hutchinson's circle and which he saw as evidence that Hutchinson and other women from her group were acting in a diabolical manner. These 'monster births' were most likely based on actual cases of miscarriage or stillbirth, but Winthrop described them in frightening terms, seeing them as proof that Hutchinson and her followers had sinned to such a degree that their very bodies had rejected the natural order. When Winthrop said that Hutchinson and her followers gave birth to monsters, he was making a claim about their religious heresy, but also about their transgression of gendered norms. According to Winthrop, Hutchinson's theological 'errors' were linked with her transgression of the proper roles of women. Therefore, she and her followers were punished by God in the form of a subversion of their reproductive powers, the most feminine aspect of their being.

Winthrop recorded his struggle against Hutchinson's heresy in his journal, which he wrote as a history of New England and was first published in the eighteenth century, as well as in a text entitled *A Short Story of the rise, reign, and ruine of the Antinomians, Familists and Libertines, that Infected the Churches of New England* (1644).[39] Winthrop's journal contains an account of the monstrous birth of one of Hutchinson's circle, Mistress Dyer. According to Winthrop, William

Dyer and his wife were both 'notoriously infected with Mrs. Hutchinson's errors', and when Mistress Dyer gave birth to a stillborn child, it was quickly buried without being seen by anyone except for the woman who reported the incident to Winthrop, the midwife Jane Hawkins who assisted at the birth, and Anne Hutchinson herself. Winthrop claimed that the child was buried so quickly because it was a monster, claiming that the midwife stated that the child was:

> of ordinary bigness; it had a face, but no head, and the ears stood upon the shoulders and were like an ape's; it had no forehead, but over the eyes four horns, hard and sharpe; two of them were above one inch long, the other two shorter; the eyes standing out, and the mouth also; the nose hooked upwards; all over the breast and back full of sharpe pricks and scales, like a thornback; the navel and all the belly, with the distinction of the sex, were where the back should be, and the back and hips before, where the belly should have been; behind between the shoulders it had two mouths, and in each of them a piece of red flesh sticking out; it had arms and legs as other children, but instead of toes, it had on each foot three claws, like a young fowl, with sharp talons.[40]

This terrifying description of the stillborn contains clear diabolical references, such as the horns, suggesting that the birth came from the devil, and that the child's mother was therefore tinged with the diabolical herself. This connection with evil was further strengthened by more testimony, claiming that when Mistress Dyer had been in labour and the monster-child died within her, the bed upon which she was lying shook and the room was filled with an awful smell to the extent that the attending women began vomiting and were forced to leave.[41] Hutchinson claimed that she hid the birth at the advice of John Cotton, who was a prominent Puritan minister. When Winthrop questioned Cotton about this advice, he said that he advised the concealment because he saw an act of providence in the fact that other women were not present to see the monstrous birth. Cotton said that had it been his child, he would have preferred to conceal the birth, and that 'he had known other monstrous births, which had been concealed, and that he thought God might intend only the instruction of the parents, and such other to whom it was known etc'.[42] Cotton fully agreed that monstrous births were a divine sign signalling to the parents that they were sinners, but unlike Winthrop he did not consider this a public sign, intended to point out the sinners for the community, but rather a private sign, intended to encourage the sinners to mend their ways.

Anne Hutchinson herself suffered a miscarriage while on trial, and Winthrop again saw this as evidence of her sinfulness and described the miscarriage as a deformed and unnatural birth in his 1644 account of the events. According to Winthrop, Hutchinson had given birth to 'not one (as Mistris Dier did) but (which was more strange to amazement) 30 monstrous births or thereabouts, at one [time]; some of them bigger, some lesser, some of one shape, some of another; few of any perfect shape, none at all of them (as farre as I could ever learne) of humane shape'.[43] Winthrop's account may sound like a sensational tabloid story, but at the time it was meant to horrify his readers and give definitive proof of Hutchinson's crimes. It presented Hutchinson as so heretical and so transgressive of her gender that even her body refused to act in an appropriately womanly manner and produce healthy children. Titillation was often used in this period in order to present providential ideas about divine punishment to a semi-literate audience, and Winthrop's exciting account of the birth fitted snugly within that tradition.[44]

Infertility and the Gendered Order

A fundamental aspect of the social pressure to have children was the centrality of childbearing to the gendered order, and through it to the social order itself. Scholars commonly state that the early modern family was a microcosm of society, and within that microcosm the man was meant to be the ruler, the wife and children his subjects.[45] The ideal woman and wife, on the other hand, was meant to be obedient, chaste and faithful.[46] Wilson argues that this interpretation lacks nuance, because conjugal authority was 'largely troubled' in this period, with no real way to enforce wifely obedience. Nonetheless, even Wilson agrees that on an ideological level conjugal authority was 'enshrined in the marriage service, affirmed in the common law, bound up with coverture and thus linked with the juridical inequality of the sexes'.[47] The ability to control one's household, and especially one's wife, was thus an important marker of masculinity, while both obedience and motherhood were important markers of femininity.[48] The ideal married woman performed her femininity by being an obedient wife and by running her household successfully, but first and foremost because she was a mother, a role which gave meaning to the work she did.[49] Fatherhood was not as central to defining masculinity as motherhood was for femininity, but it was an important component in the gendered identity of married men, who in some ways were not considered fully adult if they had no legitimate children.[50] In Sir Thomas Smith's pamphlet on the modes of rule and government in England, he described the necessary prerequisites for being considered a yeoman. According to Smith, 'commonly wee doe not call any a yeoman till he be married, and have children, and as it were have some authoritie among his neighbours'.[51] This suggests that fatherhood was an element of full membership in society as a married man, although not the only one.[52] Infertility hindered a woman's ability to perform the role of mother, and it hindered a man's ability to have a 'complete' household in which to enact his authority. Thus infertility was unsettling to the social order, and this was expressed through the repeated descriptions of infertile women as lustful, unruly and domineering, and infertile men as weak and effeminate.

Such descriptions began with the infertile body itself, which medical texts described in terms that highlight its problematic presentation of sex and gender: infertile men were described as boyish or effeminate and infertile women as dominant or masculine. 'Barren men', wrote Nicholas Fontanus in his midwifery manual, 'are commonly beardless, slow in imagination, and dull in practice, because their seed is cold, and containes not any spirit to tickle, and warm their Phantasies, but they sit like images, and are sad, and insociable.'[53] By contrast, he described fruitful men as hairy, cheerful and enjoying the company of women. Barren men were described as inherently unmanly: a smooth face evoked boys or women and they lacked any sense of action or lustfulness which could be associated with properly masculine men. Somewhat unexpectedly, hairiness was also a sign of fertility in women: 'if they [women] be rough, and full of haire, it is a signe that they are fruitful; the wiser sort of Physitians know, that much haire is an undeniable argument of much heat, and of the strength of that heat, which driveth out those fulingous humours, whereof those haires are generated'.[54] Heat was a quality associated with masculinity, but it also allowed for sexual vigour and procreation. In men, this was generally considered a good thing. In women, a moderate degree of heat was good, allowing them to experience the sexual pleasure necessary for procreation, but too much heat made them into excessively lustful barren women.[55] Women were by nature colder and moister than men, so that to be fertile a woman had to draw on some of the 'positive' male heat, but not so much so that she passed the boundaries of proper womanliness and became too hot, too masculine, and thereby both lustful and barren.[56]

These views were not merely the theoretical ruminations of medical authors. Instead, ideas about masculine, domineering infertile women and emasculated sterile men were used by real people in order to mock and criticize others. Astrological physician Richard Napier recorded a conversation with a patient who suffered from amenorrhoea and had remained childless for the two years of her marriage. Napier noted that the woman's neighbours 'mock her for a barren woman' and that the community also rebuked the couple because 'she governeth her husband & he prospereth the better, & some . . . bid him knock her down'.[57] The woman's infertility and her 'governing' behaviour appeared together because they were perceived as connected. An infertile woman was a woman who was not properly feminine, and who took over the roles of the man within the household.

Childless men were similarly presented as failing in their performance of masculinity. In September 1637, Anne Williamson and Anne Stephens were accused in the county court in the colony of Virginia for publicly insulting a man named John Waltham. A witness stated that the two women had gone to the cow pen and that they 'did in a jeering manner abuse' Grace Waltham, John's wife, by stating that her husband 'hade his Mounthly Courses as Women have' and that 'John Waltham was not able to gett a child'.[58] These insults were the sum of the accusation against Williamson and Stephens. The verdict in the case stated that these were 'most vyle and scandalous speeches', and the women were sentenced to be ducked in water, as well as to ask for the Walthams' forgiveness in front of the congregation.[59] As with New England, Virginia was still a young colony in this period, so that this case can still be seen as an example of English attitudes. The insults Williamson and Stephen chose were based on the link between effeminacy and infertility. Presumably whether the Walthams were childless or not was a matter of public knowledge. Tying the accusation to the claim that John Waltham menstruated made what might have been merely a medical matter into one that placed Waltham's very masculinity in question. Moreover, the court saw these emasculating claims as 'vyle and scandalous' enough to warrant a severe punishment involving public humiliation, and one typically associated with scolds, women who spoke up offensively in public.[60] John Waltham could not demonstrate any actual damages from these insults. He was already married, and because Williamson and Stephens did not claim that he was impotent there were no grounds for annulment.[61] Even without specific damages, however, the insult to Waltham's reputation was sufficient and required apology. Of course, if the Walthams already had children at the time, the insult was even graver, suggesting that Grace had cuckolded her husband in order to conceive.[62]

From a legal standpoint a man's first role within a marriage was to consummate it, for which he was required to be sexually potent. Once the marriage was consummated it was valid, regardless of whether it was fertile or not.[63] The legal emphasis on consummation as a test for a valid marriage has led historians to focus primarily on potency rather than fertility when looking at masculine sexuality in early modern England. Gowing argues that 'It was women . . . who were offered specific remedies to help them conceive and carry a child; the possibility of male seed failing was rarely considered.'[64] Olwen Hufton has similarly argued that 'In all European societies the blame for a failure to produce offspring was, almost without exception, laid at the feet of women,'[65] while in her study of masculinity Elizabeth Foyster similarly wrote that 'the idea that a man could be potent but sterile was not understood by early modern physicians', a view she modified in a later study with Helen Berry.[66] More recent scholarship has identified that male infertility was a more widely recognized problem in the early modern period than has previously been acknowledged.[67] Medical texts certainly acknowledged the existence of male infertility and offered remedies for it. For example, Jakob Rueff's *Expert Midwife* (1637) noted explicitly that 'sterility or barrennesse, of which wee have purposed to speak at this is present, is not onely a disability and unaptnesse of bringing forth children in women, contracted and caused by some cause that may be corrected and remedied: but in men also of ingendering and sending forth fruitfull seede'.[68] *The Compleat Midwive's Practice Enlarged* (1680) discussed enchantments after which 'the man cannot lye with his wife, or though he should, yet cannot emit the seed',[69] indicating that in some cases a man could be physically potent yet unable to impregnate his wife. In other words, infertility was not considered merely a 'women's problem' in early modern England, although they were usually the ones treated for the condition.

Because failure to consummate a marriage could lead to its annulment, it was crucial to differentiate between impotence and infertility if there was a legal issue at hand.[70] Once a marriage had been consummated, however, the fact that there were no children was not sufficient cause for such an annulment, and the marriage remained valid.[71] The distinction was thus significant if an annulment case came to court, but from a social and cultural standpoint it was not nearly as important to differentiate between cases of impotence and cases of sterility. Male infertility and impotence were not simply 'confused' in early modern England, as Angus McLaren suggests.[72] Rather, differentiating between impotence and infertility was not of significant cultural value, because it was the inability to reproduce rather than the lack of sexual performance that emasculated a man. A man who failed to impregnate his wife was a problematic man, regardless of whether his failure stemmed from an inability to perform the sexual act or from another medical problem that prevented conception. From a public standpoint the best way to identify a man who was potentially impotent was to note that his wife was not pregnant sometime after marriage, so that infertility and impotence were linked.[73]

Impotent men were subject to public ridicule in early modern Europe and its colonies.[74] In Puritan New England male impotence could be a cause for public mockery, and in some areas of Continental Europe, *charivaris* were used to publicly and communally humiliate husbands who were suspected of impotence. These involved parading the victim through the streets, sometimes on horseback, while playing loud music on pots and pans and chanting insults.[75] The English equivalent of the *charivari* was known as the skimmington, and its victims were forced to ride publicly while being accompanied by rough music and drumming. Skimmingtons did not target men who were suspected of impotence, but rather men whose wives 'wore the breeches' or took on a dominant role, especially men who were beaten by their wives. Although the wife was the aggressor in this case, it was the husband who was the target of public humiliation, because of his failure to control his wife.[76] But while the skimmington was ostensibly not linked to cuckolded men or to their fertility, the *charivari* and the skimmington both targeted men who had lost control of their household, and thus failed in their masculinity. Impotence led to a failure to satisfy one's wife, both by failing to give her sexual pleasure and by failing to impregnate her.[77] This led her to cuckold her husband, the most potent sign that a man had lost all control of his wife and was utterly dominated by her. The husband was responsible for his wife and her actions, and if she committed adultery this meant that he had failed in his duties.[78] In a similar way, if a man failed to have children soon after his marriage this was evidence of failed virility, either because of impotence or because he was infertile.

Even without a skimmington, English men could be publicly mocked for their failure to impregnate their wives, in a way that implied either impotence or infertility, but in any case placed their masculinity in question. In 1608 a libel poem circulated in writing and song in the neighbourhood of Calne, Wiltshire, which described the failure of a saddler's daughter to conceive following her marriage. The libel was brought to the attention of the local justice of the peace, in a case involving John Whittocke of Calne, a saddler, suggesting that the couple in the libel were Anne Whittocke (John Whittocke's daughter) and her husband. In 1607 Anne Whittocke married Steven Pyrkyn and they lived in the area of Calne. The manuscript copy of the libel poem was thrown into a shop on a small folded piece of paper.[79] The libel described the saddler's daughter as a young girl who rushed into marriage with a man who could not give her children.

> Oh what an earksome spite is this.
> That Sadlers of great birthe.
> No seede by anye means can have
> To florishe on the earthe.
> Maides henceforth [. . .] take yee heede
> In mariinge bee yee wise.
> Let not your husbands ficle toole
> Bee of too short a scise.[80]

If the couple in question really were Anne Whittocke and Steven Pyrkyn, their childlessness was probably short lived, as Pyrkyn fathered six children starting in 1612. The libel suggests that childless couples could be subject to public ridicule even when they had only been married for a short while, because the poem was in circulation as early as six months after Anne and Steven were married.

The libel also offers further evidence that when a couple was childless, it was not necessarily the woman who was subjected to censure and rebuke. In the libel poem, it was the husband of the saddler's daughter who was accused of having a 'tool of too short a size', which caused him to be unable to father children. This can certainly be read as a simple reference to impotence, indicating that the husband was unable to sustain an erection in order to have sexual intercourse. However, the text can also be read literally, to mean that while the couple were fully engaged in sexual activity, the husband's 'tool' was simply too short to allow for conception, a problem which was an accepted cause of fertility problems in the medical literature of the period. Massaria's *De Morbis Foeminis* discussed the impact of a short penis on conception, suggesting that 'the short *penis* [renders] men unfruitful . . . and this is the more probably reason, that the short *penis* may be more defective than the long one, because it cannot so well inject the seed into the inner parts of the womb', although the author also admitted that this was not conclusive.[81] Massaria also suggested that various deformities in the penis could prevent conception even with sexual activity. Jane Sharp, in her famous midwifery guide, similarly argued that a 'yard' that was too long or too short was unfit for generation.[82] In other words, it is possible that the libel against the saddler's daughter's husband was not claiming that he could not engage in sexual activity but that this sexual activity was not reproductive. Or rather, the libel was concerned with the fact that the husband was unable to impregnate his wife, regardless of whether the cause of that childlessness was his inability to engage in sexual activity or a medical difficulty such as an unduly short penis.

A theatrical comedy entitled *The City Bride* (1696), adapted by actor and playwright Joseph Harris from an earlier play by John Webster, offers more evidence that a man's virility was questioned when he did not father children.[83] The adaptation was performed on stage on the year of its publication, and as an urban piece and possibly one intended for a higher-class audience it suggests that these ideas circulated in a variety of social milieus. During one scene in the play, Justice Merry-man and the infertile Mrs Venter discuss her marital situation and the matter of fidelity:

> Mer. [. . .] Your Barrenness does give your Husband leave (if he please) to look for Game elsewhere.
> Mrs. Ven. Well, well Sir, tho you jeer me, and make a scorn of my Sterility.
> Mer. No, no, not I Sister, I scorn not your Sterility, nor your Husband's Virility either.
> Mrs. Ven. My Husband's Virility! Pray spare my Husband; for he has not been idle as you imagine; He may have an Offspring abroad for ought you know, that you never heard of.[84]

It is difficult to imagine a wife bragging of her husband's conquests of other women in a setting other than a comedic play. However, the scene suggests that the husband of a barren woman might be subject to a questioning of his own virility and ability to produce children, even if the wife was still considered the 'barren' one. This echoes the evidence from Napier's patient, whose husband was subject to derision because she was infertile. The play remained vague as to the exact meaning of the scorn on the husband's virility. It is possible that Merry-man was suggesting that the husband was impotent, but it could also be that his childlessness simply questioned his virility without any specific reference to sexual performance. In any case, the husband was potentially subject to scorn for the fact that he was childless. Fathering illegitimate children was frowned upon and was not considered a particularly 'manly' act in this period, and fathers of such children were subject to some social consequences to their actions (although not nearly as severe as their mothers).[85] Yet the ability of a man to father children with women other than his wife cleared him from the potential scorn associated with infertility.

The opposite story, that of a 'barren' woman who conceived after committing adultery, was more problematic, because it played into men's fear that they might raise a child who was not their own. If a woman conceived and gave birth to a child shortly after marriage, it was easier to believe that the child was her husband's, stemming from the consummation of the marriage. The longer the wait between marriage and conception, the more there was space to consider that the wife had been unfaithful, and that the child she carried was not actually her husband's child. This anxiety may have been unfounded in most cases, but this did not diminish its power. As Mark Breitenberg argues, 'The anticipation of being cuckolded... exists prior to any definitive signs of its prospect: cuckoldry anxiety rehearses a play that may never be performed since it is largely a projection of the husband's own fears translated into a story about his wife's inevitable infidelity or concupiscence.'[86] This was not only an anxiety of the individual husband towards his own wife, but rather a more widespread concern impacting the community, because the accusation that a man was a cuckold 'in terms of personal reputation would spill over into business transactions and other areas of a man's "public" persona and threaten, through such bad example, the stability of the rest of the community'.[87]

These fears, real or imaginary, found their expression in a common trope, one which found multiple cultural expressions. It was told, for example, in ballads, which focused on a young maiden whose husband would not, or could not, lie with her, leaving her wanting for both sexual satisfaction and children, and often leading her to cuckold him. The focus in these ballads was not just on the husband's failure to satisfy his wife sexually, but on the fact that in doing so he was preventing her from having children and from fulfilling the role of wife and mother. Ballads were usually written by men, so the woman's voice in these ballads is not an 'authentic' representation of women's opinions, but rather a man's view of how women thought. Such ballads therefore represent a popular public view of women's feelings, rather than the views of a specific woman. It is not one specific woman who complained that her husband cannot impregnate her, but rather a belief in a stereotypical 'young maiden' who complains that her husband would not perform his duty and by failing to perform his duty also prevented her from fulfilling her own. In the ballad *The Sorrowful Bride*, probably dating from the 1680s, a young woman complained of her husband:

> I have now been Marry'd a Twelve month and more,
> And here is a sorrow which troubles me sore;
> As having my Maiden-head now to this day;
> Is this not enough to make me run astray?
> Alas! I am almost a weary of Life,
> For to live a Maiden, tho a Marry'd wife.[88]

The ballad proceeded with a description of all of the bride's failed attempts to seduce her husband to take her maidenhead. Although the bride complained about her virginity, rather than her childlessness, at the end of the ballad she noted that her sister 'Before she full Seventeen weeks had been wed, with a Son and Daughter she was brought to bed', while the bride herself would have 'been thankful for one only son'.[89] The bride's sorrow stemmed not from her husband's failure to fulfil her sexually but from his failure to give her children through his sexual inaction. Another ballad, *The Scolding Wives Vindication* (1689), explicitly accused the husband for his wife's adultery. In this ballad it was the husband's unwillingness to copulate with his wife when she was at the prime of her reproductive capacity that led her to cuckold him. The ballad offered an explanation for the wife's actions, but it did not truly 'vindicate' her for her adultery, because she was still portrayed as scolding and unruly. At the beginning of the ballad the heroine complained that

> He's lain like a Log of Wood,
> In Bed, for a year or two,
> And wont afford me any good,
> He nothing at all would do.
> I am in my blooming Prime,
> Dear Neighbours I tell you true,

I am last to lose my Teeming Time,
Yet nothing at all he'll do.[90]

The ballad described the wife's attempt to seduce her husband, until finally the wife says:

Now let him take his ease,
And sleep while the Skye looks blue,
I have a Friend my mind to please,
Since nothing at all he'd do.[91]

The husband's lack of sexual activity and in particular his refusal to give his wife children while she was still in her prime and 'teeming' justified his wife's eventual cuckoldry of him. The cause of the women's frustrations in these two ballads technically lay in their husband's refusal or inability to engage in sexual activity with them. The crux of the problem, however, was not merely the husband's impotence but the fact that this impotence prevented the wives from having children, a fact which ultimately led the wife in the second ballad to seek other companionship.

The trope of the adulterous barren woman was neither new nor unique to early modern England. A similar idea lies at the heart of Nicolo Machiavelli's *Mandragola*, a play in which a husband is tricked into allowing another man to sleep with his wife in order to cure her supposed sterility.[92] It was not merely a powerful literary device or an amusing source of titillation, but rather an idea that had real polemic power, because tying infertility to adultery allowed authors to attack alternately the woman who had committed adultery, her husband who had failed to impregnate her or the provider of the 'cure', who assisted the wife in tricking her husband, and sometimes all three at once. It was thus used not only in jest, but also as a tool in religious and political satire. An early example of this usage appears in an anti-Catholic text from 1546, in which the author mocked 'saints' and 'monks' for cavorting with naked women under the guise of curing their infertility, noting sarcastically that 'Saynt Kentigernes disciples toke great paynes vpon them, to make barren women frutefull.'[93] This view of the actions of Catholic saints and monks was then reused in other contexts. In 1652 clergyman and historian Peter Heylyn published his *Cosmographie*, an account of various areas of the world. He included a description of the baths at Baden, in the Holy

Roman Empire, in which he both echoed earlier anti-Catholic polemic and reconfigured this polemic to fit non-religious cures for infertility:

> These Bathes are much frequented, yet not so much for health as pleasure. Their chiefest vertue is the quickning power they have upon barren women. But as the Friers used to send men whose wives are fruitless in pilgrimage to Saint Joyce, the Patroness of fruitfulness, and in the mean time to lye with their wives: so it may be with good reason thought that in a place of such Liberty as this is, the lusty and young gallants that haunt this place, produce greater operation on barren women, than the waters of the Bath itself.[94]

In the case of the previously mentioned Warming-Pan Scandal, in which Queen Mary of Modena was accused of faking the birth of a Catholic heir to the throne, this trope was used in order to attack the queen as a Catholic woman, a foreigner, and a promiscuous woman, all at once. It also served to emasculate James II and present him as a fool who had been tricked by his wife and her papal allies. The attack came in the form of a satirical poem, written as a mockery of traditional songs of thanksgiving to the Virgin. It suggested that James was unable to impregnate his wife, and that the man with whom Mary did conceive was 'Count Dada', the papal nuncio to England. According to the poem, when the Duchess of Modena, Mary's mother, died and went to heaven, she begged the Virgin to give England a son and 'putt little Oranges nose out of joynt', referring to William of Orange, the Dutch prince who would remove James II from the throne.[95] The Virgin responded by taking her own smock and asking the archangel Gabriel to carry it directly to Mary and ask her to praise the Virgin in order to 'keep the most insolent hereticks under'. James II, meanwhile was told that he

> Must be with this only to cover my daughter,
> Let him put itt upon her with his own royall hand
> Then let him goe travell and visit the land
> And the spirit of Love
> Shal descend from above,
> Though not as before in the form of a dove.
> Yet down it shall come in some likeness or other
> (Perhaps like Count Dada) and make her a mother.[96]

James, Catholic fool that he was, went on his travels, leaving his wife at Bath and allowing himself to be cuckolded and the papal nuncio's son to be proclaimed the heir—or so the poem's author claimed.

Mary of Modena treated her fertility problems by taking the waters at Bath, and claimed that she conceived a healthy child thanks to the waters. During the seventeenth century, baths gained popularity as medical sites for the elites and were particularly associated with the treatment of fertility problems. At the same time, they also became sites of social interaction, and this was often characterized as informal and even immoral.[97] The French ambassador to Charles II's court, the Comte de Gramont, described Queen Catherine of Braganza's visit to Tunbridge Wells to treat her infertility, noting that there was 'dancing every day at the queen's apartments'. The queen tried to create a more relaxed atmosphere by surpassing 'even herself in originating or sustaining new amusements. She tried to increase the natural ease of Tunbridge by dispensing with such ceremonies as were due to her.'[98] However, according to de Gramont the atmosphere may have been too relaxed and informal. 'Well may they [the waters] be called *les eaux de scandale*,' he noted, 'for they have nearly ruined the good name of the Maids and the ladies (those who are there without their husbands). It has taken them a whole month and for some more than that to clear themselves and save their honour; and it is even reported that a few of them are not quite out of trouble yet.'[99]

Because the baths had a particular association with the treatment of infertility, and were also associated with social and sexual licence, they were an excellent setting for promulgating the 'adulterous barren woman' trope. It was easy to claim that young women came to the baths to treat their infertility, only to be cured by engaging in illicit sexual activity with men other than their husbands. In 1658 John Eliot published a poem about a lady who went to Tunbridge Wells in order to 'cure her wombs sterilitie'.[100] The treatment was successful, and she gave birth to a daughter. However, this did not alleviate the shame associated with infertility, but rather 'bred about the court much mirth and laughter, because shee barren was so long before'.[101] The reason for the mockery, according to Eliot, was that it was not the water that cured the lady, but rather 'It was the pipe, rather the water cock ... it was a lusty cock o'th game'.[102] The lusty cock, of course, was a reference to a man. To make his point even clearer, Eliot proceeded by suggesting that since barrenness might prove hereditary, he hoped that the lady's 'daughter will so much wit, Early to get a cock for her cock-pit; And rather than be barren, play the whore, As her great mother hath done heretofore'.[103] Elliot's poem is merely one example of a recurring theme in the descriptions of Tunbridge Wells and Bath. Descriptions of the baths by the Earl of Rochester, Thomas Hobbes,

Jonathan Swift and others all suggested that it was not the waters of the baths that were curing barren women who went there, but rather the sexual freedom associated with being away from their husbands and in the company of young men.[104] It is interesting to note that although the lady was cured by sleeping with a man other than her husband, Elliot did not clear her from the 'taint' of being infertile, nor did he explicitly 'blame' her husband for the condition. On the contrary: he presented barrenness as a hereditary condition, one that could afflict the daughter as it had afflicted her mother. Nonetheless, it was still curable by engaging in adultery. This contradictory view was common in this literature, which saw a woman's barrenness as a kind of 'essential' quality, one which is not removed even when it is clear that the husband was the likely source of the fertility problem. This view seems to accord with the self-perceptions of women such as Mary Whitelocke, who continued to view herself as having been 'barren' for many years, with all the emotional implications of this condition, even after she easily conceived with her second husband. Nonetheless, ultimately the implications for the infertile woman's husband could not be escaped. If she needed the help of another man to conceive, it meant that her husband was unable to perform sexually at all, was unable to bring his wife the pleasure necessary for conception or was simply infertile. All of these options put the husband's virility in question.

The trope of the adulterous barren woman was used to great humorous and satirical effect, because it allowed a mockery of impotent or emasculated men while also strengthening the popular misogynist view of women as lustful and uncontrollable. Underlying this trope was the inherent masculine anxiety about being tricked into raising children that were not their own.[105] The recurrence of this theme in popular satirical literature is indicative of how pervasive these fears were and how they played out in the context of couples for whom reproduction was not straightforward. The ballad *My Dog and I* (1675) is a humorous piece about the happy exploits of a man and his 'dog', clearly a euphemism for his penis. Among his many activities, the hero of the ballad notes that that 'if Women are in distress, By reason of their Barrenness, I can a proper Prove apply, Best known unto my Dog and I'.[106] The entire ballad is a celebration of virility and manliness, exemplified by the free-spirited young man who goes where he pleases and does what pleases with his 'dog'. The implication is that a virile young man can easily impregnate a woman where her husband has failed, and that a young man could boast about the children he had fathered as a sign of his virility, so long as he was not overtly associated with the children. *The Dumb Lady or the Farriar* (1672), John Lacy's adaptation of a play by Molière, similarly offers a deceptively casual attitude towards the use of virile young men to cure infertility.[107] In the play, a seaman's wife goes to a physician to ask for his aid because '[she] has been married this dozen years, and I have never a child, and please you, and I would fain have a child, Sir'. The doctor suggests that the woman should send her husband to sea, as this 'often make the wife fruitful', indicating, of course, that with the husband away, the wife could find another lover. The doctor even goes so far as to prescribe 'a lusty Wine-porter, and he shall be thy gallant'. The wife indicates that she has tried this solution, trying 'your gallant, and your top-gallant, and your top and top-gallant, and all will do no good, Sir'. The word 'gallant' could refer to a young man who would give the woman the appropriate attentions, but it was also a nautical term describing different parts of the mast on a ship (no doubt meant as phallic symbols) and so was appropriate for the wife of a seaman. The doctor finally tells the seaman's wife to 'go try the main-yard too; and if that fail thee, thou'rt a barren woman of a certain; but come I'th'evening to me, after a glass of Wine I may have something to help thee'.[108] The main-yard is, of course, another play on words: it refers to the main mast, but a yard is also a penis. The anti-Catholic trope of the priest who attempts to 'cure' women of their barrenness was replaced here by a lecherous doctor who offers a similar service. Lacy's play implied that a barren woman might easily be cured by simply trying another sexual partner, suggesting that her husband was insufficient for the job. For Lacy's doctor, only after a woman tried multiple partners and failed to conceive could she be considered truly a 'barren woman'. Of course when the seaman's wife in the play admits to having tried 'the gallant and the top gallant…' she actually admits to being not only adulterous but also lustful and promiscuous, reifying the stereotype of women in general, and barren women in particular, as sexually immoral.

My Dog and I and *The Dumb Lady* presented a lighter view of adultery, one whose main target of ridicule is the cuckolded husband. Another satirical work by Charles Gildon, *The postboy robd of his mail* (1692), makes the link between infertility and adultery into a more insidious plot, one in which a lustful woman uses the excuse of infertility in order to receive 'permission' to cuckold her husband.[109] The work was presented as a collection of letters which were robbed from the post, with responses from those who have found the letters, although of course the letters themselves are fictional and were meant to elucidate various social 'types'.

Letter XIX was ‘from a barren Woman to a Doctor to desire his Advice what to do to Conceive’. In the letter, the woman writes that she has no children from her husband, which causes them both a great deal of dissatisfaction, particularly because the husband has no heirs. However, rather than merely seeking cure for herself, the woman suggests that ‘’tis his fault tho ‘having had the same Fate with a former Wife’.[110] One of the commentators suggests in response that ‘Ladies that have try’d Remedies for this [. . .] have generally found the change of Bed fellows more beneficial than the Bath or Wells’.[111] The other commentators suggest that the lady seems to agree with this view by stating that the problem was with her husband, thus ‘furnishing herself [. . .] with a good Plea for Cuckolding her Husband . . . If a Woman [. . .] have a mind to a thing, she’ll soon find a Reason to justifie it, as well as a opportunity to effect it’.[112] The woman in Gildon’s letter was a cultural stereotype, desiring to become a mother primarily because she is not one, and finding false justifications to allow her to cuckold her husband and to present a child not his own as his heir.[113]

Conclusion

Dror Wahrman cautions the cultural historian against relying on a ‘weak collage’, a theme that recurs within one or two connected cultural spheres, which the historian then imagines to be of cultural significance. In order to counter this risk, Wahrman suggests that the historian begin by looking for evidence of a similar idea or concept over a wide range of disparate spheres.[114] The negative descriptions of infertile men and women in early modern England appear to recur in precisely such diverse contexts. Religious literature suggested that infertility was a punishment for sins, and popular ballads reiterated the same idea. In daily conversations women claimed that childlessness or miscarriages were a sign of immorality, and mocked a barren woman for her infertility together with her dominant behaviour toward her husband. More dramatically, woman who were perceived not only as sinners but as transgressing natural feminine roles were described as giving birth to deformed and monstrous stillbirths, in both literary and ‘historical’ narratives. Infertile men, real and fictional, were described as effeminate and emasculated. And over and over, in multiple contexts and within differing social classes and locations, the story emerged of the lustful barren woman who, faced with a weak and useless husband, chose to seek sexual pleasure elsewhere, only to present her husband with a child not his own.

Together, these multiple iterations of a similar idea suggest that infertility was understood as a social problem, one that caused discomfort and was unsettling to the social order. Although many men and women never married, at an ideological level, early modern society was built on the idea of a family in which a man and a woman lived together, each playing their own unique roles. The adherence to those roles was epitomized by the bearing of children, which were described as the primary purpose of marriage, but also served to place both husband and wife firmly within their ideal social roles. When childbearing failed, then, it threatened this social order, and created an opening for the reversal of roles and an expression of anxieties about paternity. The recurring expression of these anxieties does not indicate that actual infertile women routinely attempted to sleep with men other than their husbands, nor does it imply that infertile people all faced mockery rather than sympathy and support. Indeed, it is clear that infertility was also viewed as a trying personal tragedy invoking advice and assistance. Yet the recurrence of these negative tropes, and the fact that they did not remain within literature or guidebooks, but rather appeared (with unknown frequency) in actual conversations between people of varying social class, indicates that it was part of the social world that infertile couples inhabited, and that it could impact their experience of their own fertility problems, making them more difficult to bear.

Notes

1. *A True Narrative of the Proceedings at the Sessions-House in the Old-Bayley, at a Sessions There Held on the 1st and 2nd of June, 1677* (London: Printed for D.M., 1677), pp. 4–6. The case has also been cited in Samuel S. Thomas, 'Early Modern Midwifery: Splitting the Profession, Connecting the History', *Journal of Social History* 43, no. 1 (2009): 119.
2. *The Mistaken Mid-Vvife, or, Mother Mid-Night Finely Brought to Bed* (London: Printed for F. Coles T. Vere J. Wright and J. Clarke, 1674).
3. *A True Narrative of the Proceedings at the Sessions-House in the Old-Bayley, 1st and 2d of June, 1677*, p. 6.
4. *The Mistaken Mid-Vvife.*
5. *A True Narrative of the Proceedings at the Sessions-House in the Old-Bayley, 1st and 2d of June, 1677*, p. 4.
6. Doreen Evenden, *The Midwives of Seventeenth-Century London* (Cambridge: Cambridge University Press, 1999), p. 113.
7. *A True Narrative of the Proceedings at the Sessions-House in the Old-Bayley, 1st and 2d of June, 1677*, p. 4.

8. *A Discourse of the Married and Single Life. Wherein, by Discouering the Misery of the One, Is Plainely Declared the Felicity of the Other.* (London: Imprinted for Ionas Man, 1621), pp. 25–26. This has been attributed to Roland du Jardin in Gustav Ungerer, 'Roland Du Jardin: Author of a Discourse of the Married and Single Life?', *The Library* s6-II, no. 2 (1980): 211–216; however, there is little other evidence to suggest that the attribution is correct.
9. Adrian Wilson, *Ritual and Conflict: The Social Relations of Childbirth in Early Modern England* (England: Ashgate, 2016), pp. 113–114.
10. Wilson, *Ritual and Conflict*, pp. 148–149.
11. Mark Breitenberg, *Anxious Masculinity in Early Modern England* (Cambridge: Cambridge University Press, 1996), pp. 2–5.
12. Lisa W. Smith, 'La Raillerie Des Femmes? Les Femmes, La Stérilité Et La Société En France a L'époque Moderne', in *Femmes En Fleurs, Femmes En Corps: Sang, Santé, Sexualités Du Moyen Age Aux Lumières*, ed. Cathy McClive and Nicole Pellegrin (Saint-Étienne: Publications de l'Université de Saint-Étienne, 2010), pp. 203–220.
13. Kathryn R. McPherson, '"My Deare Sister": Sainted Sisterhood in Early Modern England', in *Sibling Relations and Gender in the Early Modern World: Sisters, Brothers and Others*, ed. Naomi J. Miller and Naomi Yavneh (Aldershot: Ashgate, 2006).
14. McPherson, '"My Deare Sister": Sainted Sisterhood in Early Modern England', p. 184.
15. Ulinka Rublack, 'Pregnancy, Childbirth and the Female Body in Early Modern Germany', *Past & Present*, no. 150 (1996): 87. Anthony Fletcher, 'The Protestant Idea of Marriage in Early Modern England', in *Religion, Culture, and Society in Early Modern Britain: Essays in Honour of Patrick Collinson*, ed. Patrick Collinson, Anthony Fletcher and Peter Roberts (Cambridge: Cambridge University Press, 1994). Patricia Crawford, *Blood, Bodies, and Families in Early Modern England* (Harlow: Pearson/Longman, 2004), p. 83.
16. Abraham Wright, *A Practical Commentary or Exposition Upon the Pentateuch* (London: Printed by G. Dawson, for Tho. Johnson, 1662), p. 31.
17. *The English Midwife Enlarged* (London: Printed for Thomas Sawbridge, 1682), p. 185.
18. Alessandro Massaria and Robert Turner, *De Morbis Foemineis, the Womans Counsellour: Or, the Feminine Physitian* (London: Printed for John Streater, 1657), p. 102, likely added by the translator, as it does not appear in the original: Alexander Massaria, *Prælectiones De Morbis Mulierum, Conceptus Et Partus* (Lipsiæ, 1600).
19. Richard Bunworth, *The Doctresse* (London: Printed by J.F. for Nicolas Bourne, 1656), p. 55.

20. Robert Johnson, *Enchiridion Medicum, or, a Manual of Physick* (London: Printed by J. Heptinstall for Brabazon Aylmer, 1684), p. 245.
21. Daphna Oren-Magidor, 'From Anne to Hannah: Religious Views of Infertility in Post-Reformation England', *Journal of Women's History* 27, no. 3 (2015): 86–108.
22. Johnson, *Enchiridion Medicum*, p. 245.
23. Gowing, *Common Bodies*, p. 114–115.
24. Miranda Chaytor, 'Household and Kinship: Ryton in the Late 16th and Early 17th Centuries', *History Workshop*, no. 10 (1980): 25–26.
25. For more on the role of ballads in early modern England see Angela J. McShane, *Political Broadside Ballads of Seventeenth-Century England: A Critical Bibliography* (London: Pickering & Chatto, 2011). Patricia Fumerton, Anita Guerrini and Kris McAbee, *Ballads and Broadsides in Britain, 1500–1800* (Farnham: Ashgate, 2010).
26. Anthony Fletcher, *Gender, Sex, and Subordination in England, 1500–1800* (New Haven, CT: Yale University Press, 1995), p. xx.
27. *A Ballad, Intituled, the Old Man's Complaint Against His Wretched Son* (London: Printed for F. Coles, T. Vere and J. Wright, 1663). EBBA ID: 32615, Magdalene College 1.541.
28. Anne Halkett, *The Memoirs of Anne, Lady Halkett and Ann, Lady Fanshawe* (Oxford: Clarendon Press, 1979), p. 22.
29. Donald Lupton, *Obiectorum Reductio: Or, Daily Imployment for the Soule* (London: Printed by Iohn Norton for Iohn Rothwell 1634), p. 55.
30. Julie Crawford, *Marvelous Protestantism: Monstrous Births in Post-Reformation England* (Baltimore, MD: Johns Hopkins University Press, 2005), pp. 13–14.
31. David Cressy, *Travesties and Transgressions in Tudor and Stuart England: Tales of Discord and Dissension* (Oxford: Oxford University Press, 2000), pp. 1–3.
32. J. Bondeson and A. Molenkamp, 'The Countess Margaret of Henneberg and Her 365 Children', *Journal of the Royal Society of Medicine* 89, no. 12 (1996): 711–716.
33. Hyder E. Rollins, 'The Three Hundred and Sixty Five Children', *Notes and Queries* s2-IX, no. 237 (1922), 351b–353.
34. Samuel Pepys, *The Diary of Samuel Pepys*, vol. 2 (London: Harper Collins, 1995), p. 135. Jane Sharp, *The Midwives Book, or, the Whole Art of Midwifry Discovered* (London: Printed for Simon Miller, 1671), p. 96–97.
35. *The Lamenting Lady, Who for the Wrongs Done to Her by a Poore Woman, for Hauing Two Children at One Burthen, Was by the Hand of God Most Strangely Punished* (London: For Henry Gosson, 1620), EBBA ID: 20210, Magdalene College – Pepys 1.44–45.

36. Kelly Feinstein-Johnson, 'Reading Images and Texts: English Broadside Ballads and Visual Culture, 1600–1800' (Thesis, University of California, Santa Cruz, 2012).
37. Virginia DeJohn Anderson, *New England's Generation: The Great Migration and the Formation of Society and Culture in the Seventeenth Century* (Cambridge: Cambridge University Press, 1991), pp. 18–22.
38. For more on the Anne Hutchinson case see: Michael P. Winship, *The Times and Trials of Anne Hutchinson: Puritans Divided* (Lawrence: University Press of Kansas, 2005). Amy Schrager Lang, *Prophetic Woman: Anne Hutchinson and the Problem of Dissent in the Literature of New England* (Berkeley: University of California Press, 1987). Lyle Koehler, 'The Case of the American Jezebels: Anne Hutchinson and Female Agitation During the Years of Antinomian Turmoil, 1636–1640', *The William and Mary Quarterly* 31, no. 1 (1974): 55–78. Marilyn J. Westerkamp, 'Anne Hutchinson, Sectarian Mysticism, and the Puritan Order', *Church History* 59, no. 4 (1990).
39. John Winthrop, *The Journal of John Winthrop, 1630–1649*, vol. 1 (Cambridge, MA: Harvard University Press, 1996). John Winthrop, *A Short Story of the Rise, Reign, and Ruin of the Antinomians, Familists, and Libertines* (London: Printed for Tho. Parkhurst, 1692).
40. Winthrop, *The Journal of John Winthrop, 1630–1649*, p. 267.
41. Winthrop, *The Journal of John Winthrop, 1630–1649*, p. 268.
42. Winthrop, *The Journal of John Winthrop, 1630–1649*, pp. 267–268.
43. *The Antinomian Controversy 1636–8: A Documentary History*, ed. David D. Hall (Middletown, CT: Wesleyan University Press, 1968), p. 214.
44. Peter Lake and Michael C. Questier, *The Antichrist's Lewd Hat: Protestants, Papists and Players in Post-Reformation England* (New Haven, CT: Yale University Press, 2002).
45. Amussen, *An Ordered Society: Gender and Class in Early Modern England*, pp. 1–2.
46. Bernard Capp, *When Gossips Meet: Women, Family, and Neighbourhood in Early Modern England* (Oxford: Oxford University Press, 2003), pp. 3–5. Merry E. Wiesner, *Women and Gender in Early Modern Europe* (Cambridge: Cambridge University Press, 2000), pp. 13–35.
47. Wilson, *Ritual and Conflict*, p. 98.
48. Crawford, *Blood, Bodies, and Families in Early Modern England*, pp. 79–112. Linda A. Pollock, 'Childbearing and Female Bonding in Early Modern England', *Social History* 22, no. 3 (1997): 287–288. Olwen H. Hufton, *The Prospect before Her: A History of Women in Western Europe* (New York: Alfred Knopf, 1996), pp. 177–178.
49. William Gouge, *Of Domesticall Duties* (London: Printed by Iohn Haviland for William Bladen, 1622), p. 19.

50. Crawford, *Blood, Bodies, and Families in Early Modern England*, p. 113.
51. Shepard, *Meanings of Manhood in Early Modern England*, p. 74.
52. Jennifer Evans, '"They Are Called Imperfect Men": Male Infertility and Sexual Health in Early Modern England', *Social History of Medicine* 29, no. 2 (2014): 2. Helen Berry and Elizabeth A. Foyster, 'Childless Men in Early Modern England', in *The Family in Early Modern England*, ed. Helen Berry and Elizabeth A. Foyster (Cambridge: Cambridge University Press, 2007).
53. Nicolaas Fonteyn, *The Womans Doctour, or, an Exact and Distinct Explanation of All Such Diseases as Are Peculiar to That Sex* (London: Printed for John Blague and Samuel Howes, 1652), pp. 131–132.
54. Fonteyn, *The Womans Doctour*, p. 132.
55. Jennifer Evans, *Aphrodisiacs, Fertility and Medicine in Early Modern England* (London: Royal Historical Society, 2014), p. 53.
56. The promiscuity of infertile women was sometimes presented as a simple fact, as in: Ortensio Landi and Alain Chartier, *Delectable Demaundes, and Pleasaunt Questions, with Their Seuerall Aunswers*, ed. William Painter (London: By Iohn Cawood for Nicholas Englande, 1566), p. 2. Robert Basset, *Curiosities: Or the Cabinet of Nature* (London: Printed by N. and I. Okes, 1637), pp. 13–14.
57. Gowing, *Common Bodies*, p. 114.
58. *County Court Records of Accomack-Northampton, Virginia, 1632–1640* (Washington, DC: American Historical Association, 1954), p.85.
59. *County Court Records of Accomack-Northampton, Virginia, 1632–1640*, p. 88.
60. David E. Underdown, 'The Taming of the Scold: The Enforcement of Patriarchal Authority in Early Modern England', in *Order and Disorder in Early Modern England*, ed. Anthony J. Fletcher (Cambridge: Cambridge University Press, 1985).
61. Clara Ann Bowler, 'Carted Whores and White Shrouded Apologies: Slander in the County Courts of Seventeenth-Century Virginia', *The Virginia Magazine of History and Biography* 85, no. 4 (1977): 411–426.
62. One genealogy site claims that John and Grace Waltham had three sons, the first of which, also John, was born in about 1637, but there is no source given for this information and I have been unable to find confirmation in parish records. It is possible that the Walthams were not childless at this time, or that Grace Waltham was already pregnant.
63. Macfarlane, *Marriage and Love in England*, p. 61.
64. Gowing, *Common Bodies*, p. 114.
65. Hufton, *The Prospect before Her*, p. 177.
66. Foyster, *Manhood in Early Modern England* 69. Berry and Foyster, 'Childless Men in Early Modern England'.

67. Evans, '"They Are Called Imperfect Men": Male Infertility and Sexual Health in Early Modern England'. Catherine Rider, 'Men and Infertility in Late Medieval English Medicine', *Social History of Medicine* 29, no. 2 (2016): 245–266.
68. Jakob Rueff, 'Book 6', in *The Expert Midwife, or an Excellent and Most Necessary Treatise of the Generation and Birth of Man* (London: Printed by E. Griffin for S. Burton, 1637), pp. 11–12.
69. *The Compleat Midvvife's Practice Enlarged* (London: Printed for Nathaniel Brooke, 1659), p. 20.
70. Gouge, *Of Domesticall Duties*, p. 182.
71. Macfarlane, *Marriage and Love in England*, p. 61. Jack Goody, *The Development of the Family and Marriage in Europe* (Cambridge: Cambridge University Press, 1983), p. 190.
72. Angus McLaren, *Impotence: A Cultural History* (Chicago: University of Chicago Press, 2007), p. xiii.
73. Evans, *Aphrodisiacs, Fertility and Medicine in Early Modern England.* On male impotence and sterility in the same period in France, see: Lisa Smith, 'Imagining Women's Fertility before Technology', *Journal of Medical Humanities* 31, no. 1 (2010), pp. 76–77.
74. McLaren, *Impotence*, pp. 58–75.
75. Thomas A. Foster, 'Deficient Husbands: Manhood, Sexual Incapacity, and Male Marital Sexuality in Seventeenth-Century New England', *The William and Mary Quarterly* 56, no. 4 (1999): 734–735. Natalie Zemon Davis, *The Return of Martin Guerre* (Cambridge, MA: Harvard University Press, 1983), pp. 20–21.
76. Martin Ingram, 'Ridings, Rough Music and the "Reform of Popular Culture" in Early Modern England', *Past & Present*, no. 105 (1984): 79–113. Amussen, *An Ordered Society: Gender and Class in Early Modern England*, p. 118. Wilson, *Ritual and Conflict*, 116–117.
77. Sara F Matthews-Grieco, ed. *Cuckoldry, Impotence and Adultery in Europe* (Aldershot: Ashgate, 2014), pp. 1–2.
78. Foyster, *Manhood in Early Modern England*, p. 67.
79. *Libel of the Saddler's Daughter*, WSRO A1/110 1608E 136a-36b.This was transcribed by Rosalind Conklin-Hays, co-editor Records of Early English Drama [REED]: Wiltshire as part of that project. I would like to thank Rosalind Conklin-Hays for bringing the libel to my attention and providing detailed information about it.
80. *Libel of the Saddler's Daughter.*
81. Massaria and Turner, *De Morbis Foemineis*, p. 107. Evans, *Aphrodisiacs, Fertility and Medicine in Early Modern England*, pp. 83–85.
82. Sharp, *The Midwives Book*, pp. 22–23.

83. Joseph Harris and John Webster, *The City Bride, or, the Merry Cuckold* (London: Printed for A. Roper and E. Wilkinson and R. Clavel, 1696).
84. Harris and Webster, *The City Bride*, p. 4.
85. Amussen, *An Ordered Society: Gender and Class in Early Modern England*, pp. 112–113. Richard Adair, *Courtship, Illegitimacy and Marriage in Early Modern England* (Manchester: Manchester University Press, 1996). Johanna Rickman, *Love, Lust, and License in Early Modern England: Illicit Sex and the Nobility* (Aldershot: Ashgate, 2008). Alan Macfarlane, 'Illegitimacy and Illegitimates in English History', in *Bastardy and Its Comparative History: Studies in the History of Illegitimacy and Marital Nonconformism in Britain, France, Germany, Sweden, North America, Jamaica, and Japan*, ed. Peter Laslett, Karla Oosterveen and Richard Michael Smith (Cambridge, MA: Harvard University Press, 1980).
86. Breitenberg, *Anxious Masculinity in Early Modern England*, p. 5.
87. Matthews-Grieco, ed. *Cuckoldry, Impotence and Adultery in Europe*, pp. 1–2.
88. *The Sorrowful Bride; or, the London Lasses Lamentation for Her Husbands Insufficiency* (London: Printed for R. Kell, 1687). EBBA ID: 21258, Magdalene College Pepys 3.244.
89. *The Sorrowful Bride.*
90. *The Scolding Wives Vindication: Or, an Answer to the Cuckold's Complaint* (London: Printed for P. Brooksby. J. Deacon. J. Blare. J. Back, 1683). EBBA ID 21801, Magdalene College Pepys 4.137.
91. *The Scolding Wives Vindication.*
92. Jacques Gélis, *History of Childbirth: Fertility, Pregnancy and Birth in Early Modern Europe* (Boston, MA: Rosemary Morris, 1991), pp. 30–31.
93. John Bale, *The Actes of Englysh Votaryes Comprehendynge Their Vnchast Practyses* (Antwerp: By S. Mierdman, 1546), p. 18.
94. Peter Heylyn, *Cosmographie in Four Bookes* (London: Printed for Henry Seile, 1652), p. 142.
95. *Satirical Poem on the Birth of the Prince of Wales*, BL Stowe MS 305, f. 86.
96. *Satirical Poem on the Birth of the Prince of Wales*, f. 86v.
97. Peter Borsay, *The Image of Georgian Bath, 1700–2000: Towns, Heritage, and History* (Oxford: Oxford University Press, 2000). Peter Borsay, *A History of Leisure: The British Experience since 1500* (Basingstoke: Palgrave Macmillan, 2006).
98. Anthony Hamilton, *Memoirs of the Comte De Gramont* (London: Folio Society, 1965), pp. 210–211.
99. Margaret Barton, *Tunbridge Wells* (London: Faber & Faber, 1937), p. 139.
100. John Eliot, *Poems, or, Epigrams, Satyrs, Elegies, Songs and Sonnets, Upon Several Persons and Occasions* (London: Printed for Henry Brome, 1658), p. 58.

101. Eliot, *Poems, or, Epigrams*, p. 58.
102. Eliot, *Poems, or, Epigrams*, p. 58.
103. Eliot, *Poems, or, Epigrams*, p. 58.
104. J.B. Firth and N. Erichsen, *Highways and Byways in Derbyshire* (England: Macmillan, 1905), p. 152. John Wilmot Rochester, *John Wilmot, Earl of Rochester: The Poems, and Lucina's Rape* (Malden, MA: Wiley-Blackwell, 2010), pp. 142–143. Jonathan Swift, *The Works of Jonathan Swift* (Edinburgh: Archibald Constable and Co., 1814), p. 237.
105. Mark Breitenberg, *Anxious Masculinity in Early Modern England* (Cambridge: Cambridge University Press, 1996), pp. 2–5. Katharine Park, *Secrets of Women: Gender, Generation, and the Origins of Human Dissection* (New York; Cambridge, MA: Zone Books, Distributed by the MIT Press, 2006), p. 25.
106. *My Dog and I* (London: Printed for F. Coles, T. Vere, J. Wright, and J. Clarke, 1674).
107. John Lacy, *The Dumb Lady, or, the Farriar Made Physician* (London: Printed for Thomas Dring, 1672), p. 31.
108. Lacy, *The Dumb Lady*, p. 31.
109. Charles Gildon and John Dunton, *The Post-Boy Rob'd of His Mail, or, the Pacquet Broke Open Consisting of Five Hundred Letters to Persons of Several Qualities and Conditions, with Observations Upon Each Letter* (London: Printed for John Dunton, 1692), pp. 89–90.
110. Gildon and Dunton, *The Post-Boy Rob'd of His Mail*, p. 89.
111. Gildon and Dunton, *The Post-Boy Rob'd of His Mail*, p. 90.
112. Gildon and Dunton, *The Post-Boy Rob'd of His Mail*, p. 90.
113. Gildon and Dunton, *The Post-Boy Rob'd of His Mail*, p. 90.
114. Dror Warhman, 'Change and the Corporeal in Seventeenth and Eighteenth Century Gender History: Or, Can Cultural History Be Rigorous?', *Gender & History* 20, no. 3 (2008): 584–602.

CHAPTER 5

Treating Fertility Problems

A significant portion of Mary Whitelocke's memoir is dedicated to describing the long years in which she struggled with infertility. Whitelocke wrote of her desire for a child and her emotional anguish, and thought a great deal about how she understood infertility as part of the divine plan. Within this long description, Whitelocke allocated only one sentence to a description of the actions she took in her attempts to conceive. 'We had been much in prayer to the lord for a child, as Hannah did,' she wrote, 'and at last the lord h[e]ard my prayer after I had taken very much phisicke and been at the waters and at the bath.'[1] Whitelocke included this description because she was writing within the genre of spiritual memoir. Her point was to guide her son's faith, not to give him the details of her treatments. Nonetheless, this sentence not only summarizes Whitelocke's years of infertility, but also the basic treatment options available to early modern couples struggling with reproductive difficulties.

First and foremost, infertility was understood within a religious framework, and Protestant couples relied on prayer and faith both to give meaning to their condition and to hope for a cure. There is also some evidence that the Catholic minority continued to rely on fertility rituals such as praying to saints and going on pilgrimages to holy sites. These practices were formally forbidden, but did not disappear after the Reformation.[2] Prayer was important, but it was seen as complementary to other forms of treatment, which might be placed in the broad category

D. Oren-Magidor, *Infertility in Early Modern England*,
Early Modern History: Society and Culture,
DOI 10.1057/978-1-137-47668-5_5

of 'physic', or medicine. This might involve treatment by university-educated physicians, but was more likely to be self-treatment, or treatment by the wide range of informal practitioners who provided care in this period. Whitelocke herself didn't elaborate on the physic she took for her fertility problems, but she did record a later incident in which her son Samuel was ill, so much so that he refused to swallow medicine or anything else. In that case, Whitelocke consulted several practitioners, and noted that 'there was a good woman [who] sent me a mediason for him, and I having 4 doctors for him, some of my friends ware against his taking of any woman's medisons'.[3] However, Samuel relented and agreed to swallow some medicine just at the moment when the woman delivered her remedy. Whitelocke saw this as an act of providence and immediately began administering the controversial treatment, which quickly brought Samuel back to health. Whitelocke could afford trained physicians and made use of them when she felt it necessary, but she did not limit her medical arsenal to what they had to offer. It is likely she did the same when it came to her fertility woes. Finally, Whitelocke differentiated between 'physic' in general and taking the waters at the baths. Water cures became increasingly popular throughout the seventeenth century for the treatment of a range of medical conditions. They became particularly associated with fertility problems after several of England's queens used them for that purpose. Medicinal bathing was still limited to a fairly small and elite social group, which could afford to take vacations specifically for this purpose. Within that group, water cures became the treatment of choice for reproductive disorders.

Just as religion and medicine complemented one another in explaining infertility, so they also functioned together in treating it. It was understood that God afflicted people with ailments, including infertility, and that God also provided the cure. Sometimes this was done through His direct intervention, but more prosaically it was done through His provision of effective medicines.[4] There was a common understanding that God revealed His truth in two ways: biblical scripture or the divine Word, and 'the Book of Nature', the type of divine truth that could be learned by observing the natural world and its rules. Medicine was a natural gift that God gave to mankind in order to allow them to survive illness.[5] Any form of physic was meant to be taken together with prayer, and indeed guidebooks to medicinal bathing often noted specific types of prayers to be used before and during the treatment.[6] Ian Mortimer argues that as the seventeenth century progressed, patients increasingly sought to replace 'spiritual physic' with paid medicine in treating serious medical conditions.[7] The evidence of fertility problems, however, suggests quite a different picture. Early modern women, even at the end of the seventeenth century, were reluctant to approach male medical practitioners to treat fertility problems, preferring instead to use 'kitchen physic', self-treatment in the home, or possibly paying female practitioners.[8] More significantly, even in the late seventeenth century, and even outside distinctly godly circles, religion played a crucial role in both the understanding and treatment of fertility problems. This may have been connected to the intense and personal religiosity of early modern women, who found particular comfort in their lives through piety and faith.[9]

Early modern patients made use of the full range of prayers, rituals and treatments available for fertility problems, choosing the options that best suited their beliefs, needs and means. Indeed, the distinction between humoral medicine, chemical medicine, sympathetic magic and other forms of cures appears to have been largely meaningless to patients, who were quite happy to try various remedies to achieve the desired result. Lisa Smith states that in early modern France there was considerable pressure on women to try every available remedy, regardless of its cost or how dangerous or unpleasant it might be.[10] There is little evidence of such explicit pressure on English women, but they were certainly no less willing to try different forms of remedies than their French counterparts.

Prayer

Scholars of the English Reformation caution us against seeing it as a revolution, a sudden change which swept away all Catholic beliefs and practices to be replaced by Protestant ones.[11] Both before and after the Reformation, men and women who suffered from fertility problems relied on their faith to help them cope with their condition and to seek treatment for it. However, the Reformation did bring about changes in the available practices for such treatment. Protestants and Catholics alike believed in the importance of prayer, and in the likelihood that prayers would be answered if God willed it, but while Catholic women could pray to the Virgin Mary and to a host of saints, Protestant women were admonished to pray only to God Himself.[12] As Tessa Watt points out, the 'post-Reformation' religion did away with many of the most obvious visual signs of Catholicism, notable among these the worship of saints, and replaced them with 'Bible-centred Protestantism', in which there were still role models and heroes, but these tended to be Biblical.[13] Thus when it came to treating fertility problems, rituals related to saints and their holy sites were replaced with direct prayers to God and a reliance on biblical role models such as Sarah and Hannah.[14]

In the late middle ages, devotional practices relating to medical conditions often involved the intercession of saints. The Church stressed that 'the saints were only intercessors whose entreaties might go unheeded'. At the same time, it also encouraged practices relating to saints by promoting the idea that such prayers and rituals had a good chance of succeeding.[15] Like most other aspects of life, reproductive matters had their own patron saints. The Virgin Mary, as the ultimate role model for mothers, was one target for women's reproductive hopes. Mary's mother, St Anne, was considered the patron saint of barren women, because there was an apocryphal belief that she had been unable to conceive without divine intervention.[16] Devotional practices involving these saints included pilgrimages, prayers and offerings, as well as a variety of relics, ampullae and other paraphernalia. Infertile women as well as those who wanted to prevent miscarriage or to have easy labour might go on pilgrimage or practise rites involving saints' statues or relics. At Walsingham in Norfolk pilgrims could purchase ampullae filled with holy water and a drop of the Virgin's milk, probably used to aid in fertility, childbirth or lactation.[17] Women could also perform other devotional acts relating to the saints. Katherine Denston, from a family of prominent fifteenth-century Suffolk merchants, commissioned a poem on the life of St Anne, meant as a talismanic entreaty to the saint to assist her in conceiving of a son (she already had a daughter, interestingly named Anne).[18] While specific saints were particularly associated with reproduction, fertility-related cures could also occur in shrines belonging to other saints. A woman visiting St Thomas Cantilupe's shrine in Hereford was cured of her infertility and conceived twins.[19] The wife of William, a knight of Lincoln, was cured of her sterility at the shrine of Thomas Becket and named her son Thomas in recognition of the saint's benefaction.[20] Catherine of Aragon, hoping to conceive of a son, went to St Frideswide's priory at Oxford to ask for the saint's assistance with her conception. St Frideswide's shrine was particularly associated with women, although not necessarily with fertility problems. Women appear twice as often as men in St Frideswide's collection of miracles.[21] In addition to saintly intercession, medieval believers had other means of gaining religious aid on reproductive matters. Invocations involving priests using crosses and holy water were used to make a marriage bed fertile and to counter sterility in both animals and women.[22] Holy Communion was also used to treat infertility, and scrolls containing protective prayers could be used as girdles to protect women during labour.[23] Miracle cures were used either in conjunction with medical treatment (by learned physicians as well as more informal medical practitioners) or after all medical intervention had supposedly failed.[24] They were not an alternative to medical treatment but worked together with it.

Before the Reformation, water cures were also ritual practices, meant to invoke specific saints connected with a specific location. Certain waters became associated with the treatment of fertility problems, such as the well at Shottery in Warwickshire, which was associated with 'women's complaints'.[25] St Frideswide's well in Binsey, Oxfordshire, was also associated with women's illnesses.[26] The well can still be seen outside St Margaret's Church on the outskirts of Oxford. Perhaps most important of the healing wells was St Winifred's well, at Holywell, north Wales. At this site the deaf regained their hearing, the blind saw again, devils were cast out, crutches were set aside and barren women became fruitful.[27] The use of these wells as holy sites by Catholics did not entirely end after the Reformation. James II visited Holywell on 29 August 1687, to entreat with St Winifred so that his wife might conceive.[28] James's Protestant opponents used this as one more source of criticism against him. One political pamphlet saw the visit to the well as a step meant to prove the future claim that Mary had given birth to a son. 'Be pleased to remember,' it noted 'that 'tis before observed, that the going to the *Bath*, and the visit to St. *Winifred's Well*, and the Present made to the *Lady*, were preparations for a Report of the *Queen's* being with Child.'[29]

Pilgrimages to holy wells were not the only form of Catholic fertility ritual that continued to be practised by some English women after the Reformation. Mary Fissell writes that 'In the later sixteenth and early seventeenth centuries, recusant women continued to employ girdles of the Virgin, wax amulets of the *agnus dei*, and other sacred objects to ensure successful childbirth.'[30] There was also a privileged group of women, England's Catholic queens, who were allowed to practise their religion openly, a fact which allows us a more detailed view of Catholic fertility rituals after the Reformation. These practices were closely connected to Continental practices, such as those used by Louis XIII and Anne of Austria.[31] In addition to prayers at Holywell, Queen Mary of Modena relied on offerings to saints, prayers and the wearing of clothes blessed in shrines in her attempt to give birth to a healthy male heir to the English throne. These attempts were fodder for anti-Jacobite propaganda, which used it to stress the 'heretic' nature of the royal couple with their Catholic beliefs, as well as the queen's foreign origin. One form this propaganda took was that of playing cards, which depicted events leading up to the Revolution of 1688 and served to justify the revolution. These cards most likely circulated in coffee shops and taverns.[32] Three of these card explicitly depicted fertility rituals: prayers to the Virgin Mary as the Lady of Loreto for the birth of a prince, the Duchess of Modena, Mary's mother, offering gold to the same statue to ensure Mary's conception, and Mary receiving a smock from Rome that had been consecrated, perhaps by being placed on the statue of the Virgin or one of the saints. The cards highlight the 'problematic triumvirate of Catholic queen consort, Virgin Mother, and maternity', which ultimately led to James II's ousting and to the constitution prohibiting not only a Catholic king, but also a Catholic consort (Figs. 5.1, 5.2 and 5.3).[33]

Given the polemic nature of these cards, it is difficult to be certain whether Mary actually performed these rituals, but they do not seem out of character for a Catholic woman seeking a cure for fertility problems. Catholic women were known to wear items which had previously been placed on the statue of a saint or of the Virgin Mary, in order to ensure a safe pregnancy.[34] France's royal family had long prayed to the Virgin for sons and went on pilgrimages to promote childbearing when faced with infertility.[35] Although the depictions in the playing cards were designed to enrage a Protestant English public, they depict Catholic rituals similar to those used by actual barren women in order to cure their condition. These practices offered infertile women a sense that there was something active they could do in order to conceive, even if medicine could offer no hope, because they could achieve miraculous results through the invocation of the saints.

The Reformation changed the available options for most women, who could no longer rely on saintly intercession of this kind. In the mid-sixteenth century, anti-Catholic authors published scathing mockeries of the miracle stories attributed to various saints and holy men. The stories of saints curing infertile women were excellent fodder for such criticism, because they relied on the same bawdy suggestions as the trope of adulterous barren women. It was simple to claim that various holy men 'cured' infertility by bedding women, rather than through any ability to channel divine powers or perform miracles. John Bale, who converted to Protestantism during Henry VIII's reign, devoted his *Actes of the Englysh*

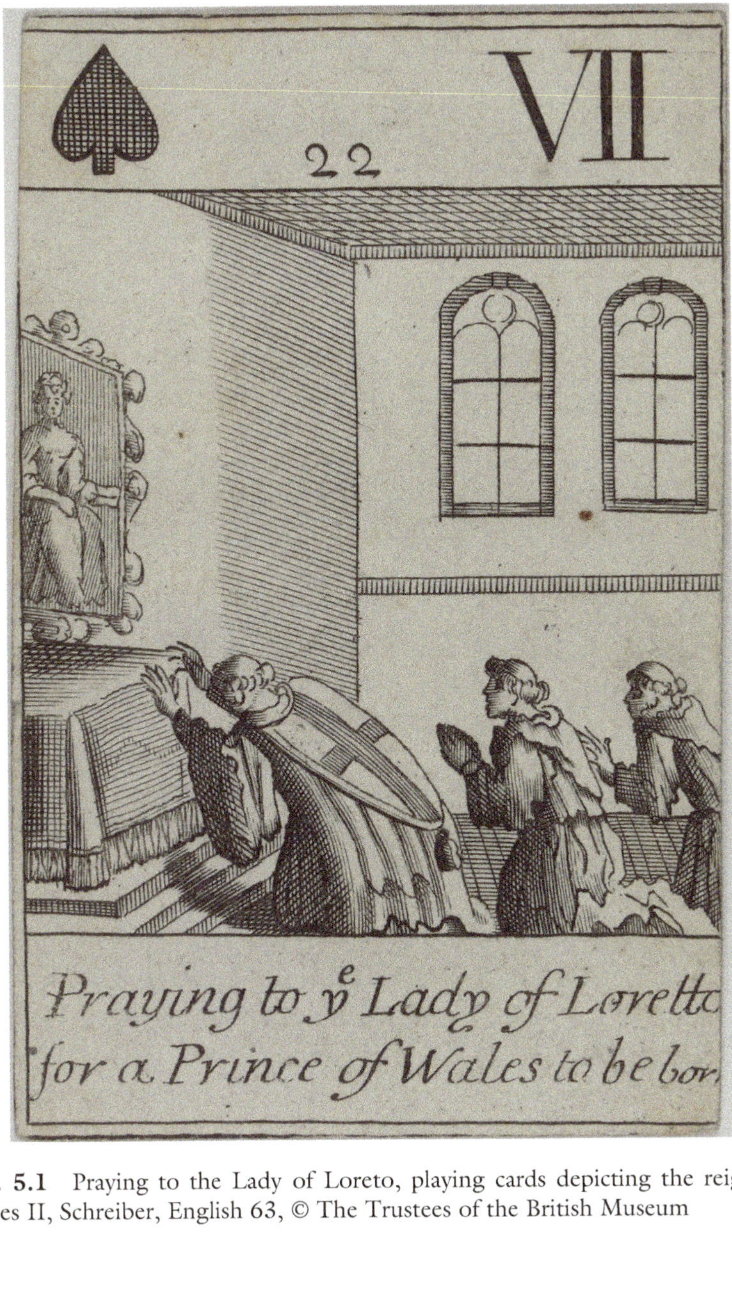

Fig. 5.1 Praying to the Lady of Loreto, playing cards depicting the reign of James II, Schreiber, English 63, © The Trustees of the British Museum

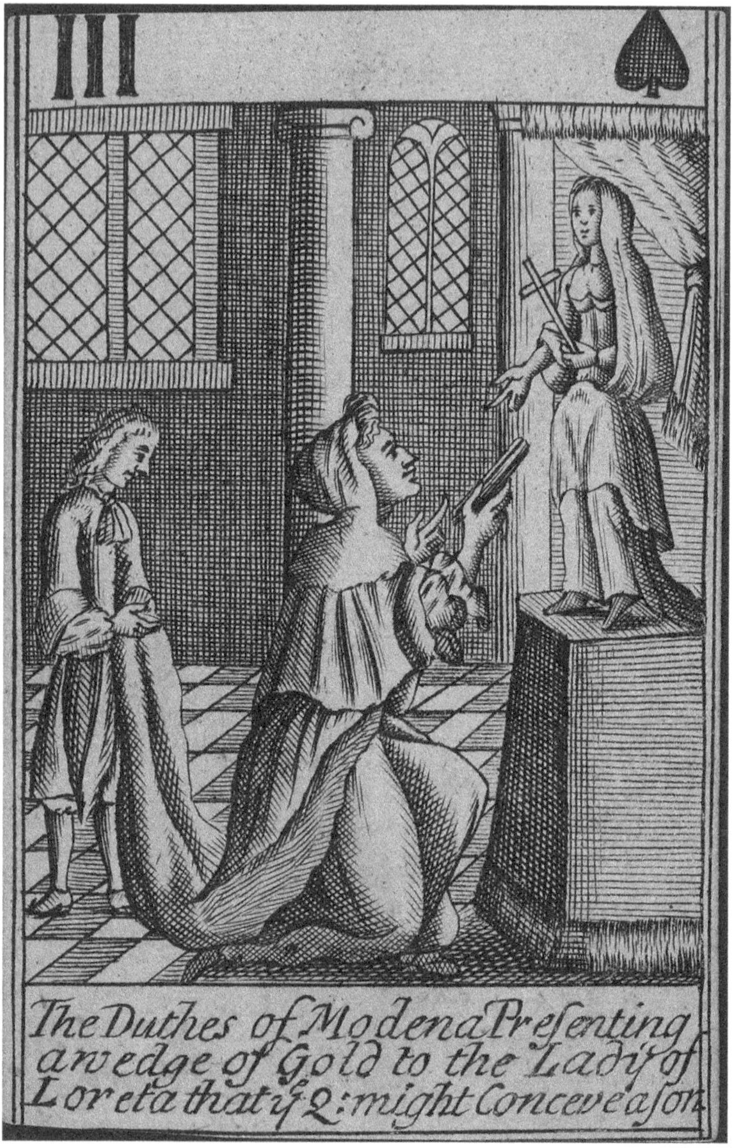

Fig. 5.2 The Duchess of Modena presents a wedge of gold to the Lady of Loreto, playing cards depicting the reign of James II, Schreiber, English 63, © The Trustees of the British Museum

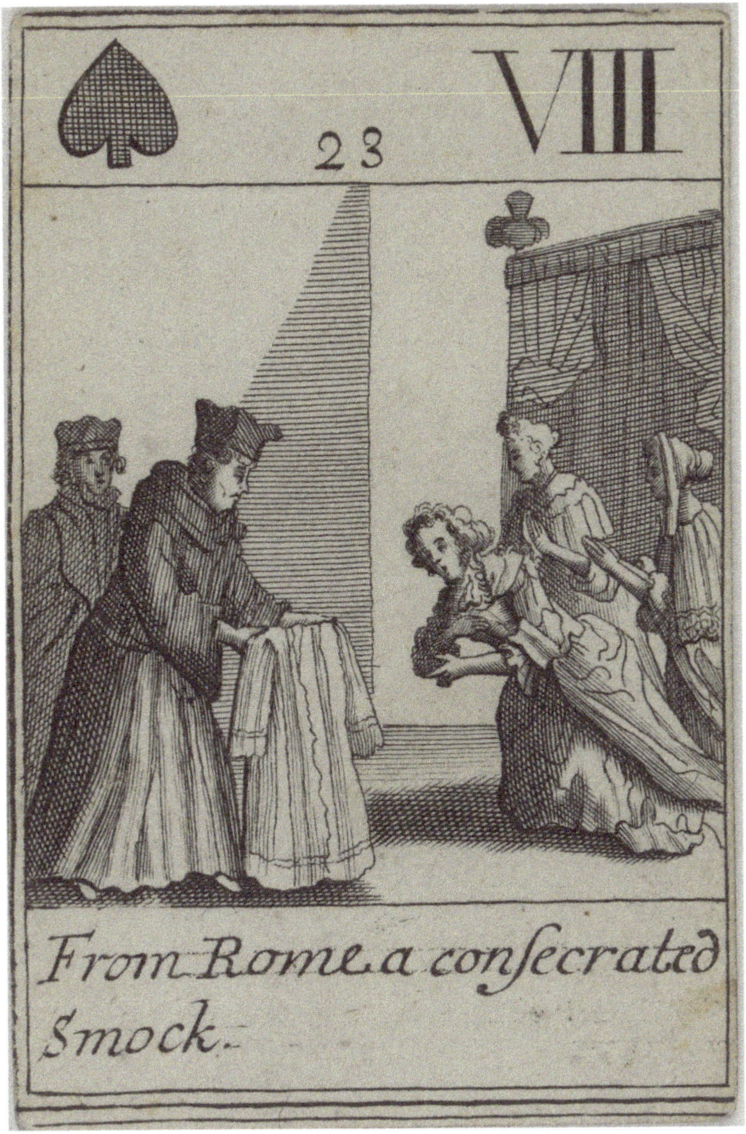

Fig. 5.3 From Rome a consecrated smock, Francis Barlow[?], the revolution, playing cards, © The Trustees of the British Museum

votaryes (1546) to the revelation of the 'false myracles' of the saints.[36] In one section, he mentioned 'Saynt *Foillanus*, an Iryshe Bishop with hys bretherne was verye famylyar and seruysable unto Saynte Gertruyde and her nonnes at *Nigella*, made dyverse barren women full gracyouslye to conceyve'.[37] Similar mockery of Catholic cures was made in a much later piece, the *Monk Unvail'd* (1678), a satirical anti-Catholic dialogue purportedly translated from a work by 'a French Papist', Jean Barrin. One of the speakers says: 'You have named one Father *Ralph*: I knew in *Averna* one of that name, whose Beads, as he said, had the vertue to cause barren women prove with Child. So that there was no barren women in any place, where that Father had been, but were advised to make use of Father *Ralph's* Beads.'[38] Like Bale, the author of the *Monk Unvail'd* at once mocks Catholic practices and accuses Catholic clergymen of immoral behaviour. An innocent reading of the text would suggest that Father Ralph cured barren women using the power of his rosary beads, but of course the satirical tone of the text implied that the 'beads' in question were actually his testicles.

Anti-Catholic rhetoric discredited a belief system that allowed for the idea of regular miraculous intervention into daily life and gave believers the ability to ask saints for intercession on their behalf, but Protestant preachers and theological writers also tried to offer their believers some sort of alternative that would fulfil a similar purpose.[39] Believers needed to feel that despite the lack of saintly intercession there was still hope even in situations that felt hopeless, and that they had some method of applying God's power to their own lives. In order to achieve this, Protestant clergy increasingly focused on the idea of God's omnipotence and divine providence—that God was an active deity, one who took complete interest in the lives of the believers and without whom nothing happened in the world.[40] God controlled everything that happened both in the universe in general and for each person in particular, and this included not only regular occurrences but also irregular ones, such as the punishing of the wicked on the one hand and the apparently miraculous—such as curing a barren woman—on the other. God's intervention could be sought by those who had faith and who prayed earnestly, although faith and prayer were not direct avenues for achieving a result, because even those who promoted prayer stated that there was no guarantee that prayers would be answered.[41] Nonetheless, prayer to God offered believers a ritual practice with which to seek divine aid for their problems that served a similar function to Catholic rites requesting intercession.

Prescriptive religious literature advised women to learn from the examples of the biblical barren women Sarah, Rachel and Hannah and to pray modestly and earnestly for a child.[42] Women who wanted to emulate Hannah directly could find the exact biblical text of her prayer to God for a child as well as her prayer of thanksgiving after having a child in Thomas Bentley's *Monument of Matrons* (1582).[43] This was essentially a collection of prayers and other texts supposedly written by various women both historical and contemporary, which was meant to give religious guidance to women in various aspects of their lives. However, Hannah's prayers were not simply listed in order to recount her story. Instead they were repurposed for general use by women who wanted to conceive, as is evident from the fact that they were indexed under the heading 'Against barrennesse'.[44] Another religious guide, Samuel Hieron's *Helpe Unto Devotion*, was published in numerous editions between its first appearance in 1608 and at least until 1650. It became one of the most popular works of piety in seventeenth-century England.[45] From its second edition, the book contained a prayer for barren women, in which she was explicitly directed to view herself in the context of the Biblical stories. The prayer's heading was: 'Som barren Hannah, or childlesse Elizabeth, desiring to bee blessed with fruite of bodie, prayeth thus.'[46] This heading created a direct connection between the barren woman reading the book and using the prayer and her Biblical role models. Hieron encouraged women reading his book to consider the examples of holy women who had been afflicted with infertility and who were cured, seeing their stories as proof both that God could cure them and that they should not see their infertility as a sign that God did not love them or had abandoned them.[47] They were to ask God to

> Make me (O good God) as sensible of my spirituall defects, as I am of these bodilie inflictions. And as it is reported of thee in the word, that thou makest the barren woman to dwell with a familie, and to be a joyfull mother of children, so make mee (I humbly crave of thee in Jesus Christ) an example of they mercy herein. Let mee bee as the fruitfull Vine on the walles of my husband's house, and let (at the least) one Olive plant spring out from mee, to stand about his table. The fruite of the wombe is they reward, of thee alone doe I desire it, from they mercie onely doe I expect it.[48]

Prayer was thus presented as an active tool for infertile women to ask for a child. The *Ornaments for the Daughters of Zion* (1692) by New England minister Cotton Mather also contained a discussion of infertility that utilized biblical examples in order to prescribe how women should behave in the face of reproductive problems. According to Mather, a woman should expect and desire to have children after marriage because they are a blessing. However, if she did not conceive, she need not see this as an insurmountable obstacle.[49] Rather, she had a direct role model in the Bible, that of Hannah. Like Hannah, she could pray to God and know that He had the power to make her fruitful. Mather also stated what barren women should not do, using Rachel as a negative role model, because of her impatience and her demands that she must have a child or else she would die. The consequences of such improper demands on God might be severe, according to Mather. 'But she [the barren woman] will not Impatiently long,' he wrote, 'like *Rachel, Give me Children or else I Dy*, Lest she *Dy* by her having of those *Children*.'[50]

As Chapter 2 demonstrated, devout infertile women took this advice to heart, and saw prayer as a central tool to deal with infertility and essentially to 'treat' it, by asking God to cure their condition.[51] Whitelocke's memoirs and Margaret Hoby's diary indicate that faith and prayer were not used instead of other methods of treatment, but rather worked together with them in order to provide a complete approach to treating fertility problems. The belief was that remedies and cures were divine gifts and all healing only took place if God willed it, so that praying for a child worked together with taking home remedies, seeking advice from physicians and consulting other medical practitioners. Whatever treatment worked, it did so only because it was part of a divine plan.

Physic

The early modern medical marketplace was large and varied, and this variety was as true for fertility problems as for all other conditions.[52] As with most ailments in this period, the first recourse for fertility problems was 'kitchen physic'. This was knowledge that was collected by laypeople (laywomen especially) and was used in order to create remedies and cures in a home setting, rather than seeking the advice of paid medical practitioners.[53] While kitchen physic was the basic form of treatment for almost anything in this period, women suffering from fertility problems were particularly reluctant to consult male practitioners and preferred to deal with their condition by getting advice from their female peers, or perhaps from female practitioners. They usually consulted male practitioners only when their condition was particularly long-lasting or severe, when they were suffering from dangerous complications from a miscarriage or stillbirth, or when their fertility problems were only part of a wider medical condition for which they were seeking treatment.[54] It was also not uncommon for patients to use multiple forms of treatment at the same time, relying on home remedies, physicians and other practitioners all at once.[55]

Broadly speaking, fertility patients in this period were women. Even when men asked for advice about having children, they were usually doing so with the intent of treating their wives, rather than taking any cure themselves. While medical texts recognized the existence of male infertility, there is little evidence of men seeking advice for their own fertility problems. In theory men could be infertile, but in practice infertility was almost always 'blamed' on women.[56] Jennifer Evans notes that fertility medicines were offered to men, and that surgeons were concerned about fertility when dealing with hernias, but not actual cases in which male patients sought fertility advice from a practitioner.[57] The best known case of a man seeking fertility advice is that of Samuel Pepys, who asked a group of women at a party for advice on his childlessness.[58] He wrote about this event in a diary entry on 26 July 1664, noting that he had attended a party in honour of the 'gossips' who had attended at the birth of his godchild. Pepys noted having sent 'a dozen and a half bottles of wine' to the event, bottles which no doubt aided in creating the very 'merry' atmosphere at the dinner. When the women rose from the table, Pepys decided to join them, 'ne'er a man but I', and 'began discourse of my not getting of children and prayed them to give me their opinions and advice', advice which the women dispensed 'freely and merrily'.[59] The gossips offered ten pieces of advice, of which Pepys noted that they were particularly serious about the advice to drink sage juice, to keep the 'stomach warm and back cool' and to engage in sexual activity 'when we had most mind to it'. More light-hearted advice included avoiding restrictive clothes, eating late dinners and hugging his wife gently.[60] The advice the women gave consisted of remedies for Pepys himself, remedies for his wife Elizabeth and advice for the couple to follow together. They made no assumption about who was 'at fault' for the fertility problem. While this is an interesting case, it does not seem to be highly representative of the usual practice of couples with fertility problems, as little other evidence exists of men seeking treatment for infertility. This incident is the only time Pepys recorded seeking medical advice for childlessness, and it is telling that he consulted a group of laywomen who were essentially dispensing 'kitchen physic' rather than any kind of 'professionals'.[61]

When home remedies were not successful over a period of time, or the stakes were particularly high, patients sought help from external practitioners.[62] These ranged from university-educated physicians or licensed surgeons, who practised with official approval, to unlicensed practitioners such as apothecaries (who were supposed to dispense medicines but not to diagnose or treat illness), astrologers, purveyors of patent medicines and cure-alls, and a variety of male and female healers of all classes and kinds.[63] The remedies themselves varied in type and in the rationale by which they were expected to work, whether they were prescribed by a paid practitioner or made at home using a private recipe collection. Most medical advice in this time was loosely based on Galenic principals and was aimed at balancing the humours. Chemical medicines were also growing in popularity, and were usually provided by 'professionals' because they were difficult to make at home.[64] There were various kinds of magical treatments, from obscure alchemical procedures that may never have been used to actually treat a real case to potions and spells provided by 'wise women' and popular healers.[65] It is tempting to categorize these treatments according to the rationale by which they functioned, but such categorization would not have made much sense to the patients themselves. Private medical recipe collections contained purely humour-based medicines side by side with magical cures. The same was true for published medical manuals written by licensed physicians. Women circulated astrological advice at the same time as they exchanged herbal recipes for reproductive cures. Physicians prescribed water cures together with other forms of treatment. There was usually little attempt to explain the mechanics of how treatments worked and more focus on their efficacy and uses. By and large, early modern fertility patients chose those treatments that they could afford and that they believed were efficacious, based on previous experience or the advice of trusted acquaintances. They did not much care if the cure was supposed to work by balancing the excess humours, by sympathetic magic or by some 'occult quality' that had no clear explanation.[66] It is therefore more meaningful to examine who provided treatment and what options they offered, looking at self-treatment in the home, treatment by 'professional' practitioners of all kinds, water-cures as a distinct social/medical option that emerged during this period, and religion not only as a general explanatory model for illness and disease in which patients were healed only if God willed it, but also as a set of specific rituals and processes that were intended to assist in reproduction.

Much of our information about how people treated fertility problems in the home comes from handwritten medical recipe books, which were kept by both men and women, but were considered particularly important for women who managed a household. Women were expected to provide healing services for those in their household, and upper-class women often administered medical aid to the poor as a form of Christian charity.[67] The remedies and medical recipes that such women used in their practice were received from friends and relatives and copied down from advice or prescriptions received from medical practitioners. In some cases they were also copied down from printed medical manuals or collections of recipes.[68] Most of the recipes were based on the theory of the humours, meaning that they were expected to function in a way that would moderate the temperament of the body or aid in balancing the humours. However, such recipes were based on a very practical understanding of humoral theory: that consuming products that were hot and dry, for example, would counteract a condition that stemmed from excess cold and moisture. The recipes did not contain any theoretical explanation about how they functioned, nor were they placed in the context of an overall change in regimen that was meant to be a part of humoral treatment.[69] Medical recipe collections belonging to men might contain some reproductive recipes, but they were more common in women's recipe collections, although even there they did not make up the majority. Common recipes deal with fevers, agues, palsy, cuts, wounds, cancer and various forms of pain. Most medical recipe books written by women did contain some cures for reproductive difficulties, including recipes for promoting conception, preventing miscarriages, assisting in labour (including that of stillborn babies) and bringing on menstruation. It has been suggested that the latter recipes were actually meant to be used as abortifacients rather than for the promotion of fertility.[70] Such an interpretation seems problematic given the fact that menstrual disorders were considered one of the causes of fertility problems, as well as the fact that some recipes of this kind were meant to be used on a monthly basis.[71] Recipes 'to bring on the flowers' may have been used as abortifacients, but they were undoubtedly also meant to treat amenorrhea as a cause of infertility as well as a condition which was considered hazardous to a woman's health and potentially even fatal.[72]

Recipes in handwritten collections were sometimes copied from printed manuals, indicating that women read vernacular medical texts and found them useful. Some women even commented on the sources they copied and took notes from their reading.[73] While this was a popular practice, it was not universally approved, because physicians worried that through ignorance or merely taking recipes out of context, patients would use the advice incorrectly. Physician James Primrose criticized women for taking 'their remedies out of English books or else make[ing] use of such as are communicated to them by others, and then they think they have rare remedies for all diseases', a matter which Primrose found particularly objectionable because it meant that they were not following Galen's advice of tailoring the recipe to the particular patient.[74] From the point of view of traditional Galenic medicine, Primrose's criticism was not without merit. The humoral medicine of the university-trained physician theoretically promoted a comprehensive approach to health, an overall regimen of diet, exercise and conduct which was supposed to maintain the body in a balanced state of health, or restore it to health when the balance was disturbed. Recipe books offered general remedies that could be used by any patient to treat a condition. This focus on remedies rather than on more holistic medical advice was driven by the preferences of the patients themselves, who usually preferred the use of a remedy to complicated and often costly changes in regimen.[75] Despite the fact that fertility problems were often attributed to lifestyle factors such as diet or exercise, most of the remedies which women collected were in the form of 'cures', meaning a specific medication to be taken to treat a particular condition, without necessarily requiring a change in habits. Given that medical texts implied that infertility was caused by life choices that were immoral or sinful, such as excessive sexual activity or gluttony, the focus on remedies rather than holistic changes may not have been merely a matter of convenience, but also to some extent a rejection of a narrative that blamed the patient for her fertility problems.

Many fertility recipes relied on the use of common ingredients such as wild herbs and garden plants, including sage, rosemary, mugwort, leeks and parsley.[76] One recipe which appeared in several collections called for the use of a plant which 'groweth by the sea side'.[77] This was probably eringium, or sea holly, which was an inexpensive and available remedy.[78] Many recipe books contained a combination of medical and cookery recipes, sometimes with little distinction between them, so it is hardly surprising that many reproductive recipes also used common food ingredients. Elizabeth Jacobs, a seventeenth-century recipe collector, listed a recipe to aid conception in which the preparer should 'seeth the fish called a Trout in goat milke, and give it the party to drink when she goes to bed'.[79] Johanna St John's many reproductive recipes included a broth made of veal and mutton, while Katherine Palmer suggested the use of a drink made from '3 quarts of milk and the whites of 2 eggs beaten' to prevent miscarriage.[80] One sensible recipe in an anonymous collection suggested that when a pregnant woman wanted to avoid giving in to her cravings, she should 'take a wine glass of spring water, drinke it, and if that will not cure, another'.[81] The use of fairly commonplace ingredients meant that recipes could be used by people from all social classes, although it is difficult to track the circulation of this advice among illiterate women.

In addition to common and local ingredients, some recipes used more expensive spices, many of them imported from Asia, such as cinnamon, cloves and galangal (a form of ginger). Despite their exotic origins, by this period many of these ingredients would have been relatively common in wealthier households and were used quite regularly in cookery recipes as well as medicinal ones.[82] There is little indication that expensive or exotic ingredients were considered more effective than common garden herbs. John Davall's recipe collection included 'a good thing to make a woman fruitfull', which he attributed directly to 'the romishe queen', referring to Henrietta Maria, wife of Charles I. Despite the royal pedigree of this recipe, it used nothing more than wild sage boiled in water or wine.[83] Many of the recipes in these collections used both common garden-variety ingredients and exotic spices in the same recipe. For example, one of Aletheia Talbot Howard's recipes to aid with conception called for a combination of spices such as ginger, cinnamon, nutmeg and cloves, with more prosaic plants such as sage, thyme and rosemary.[84] The primary distinction was whether a remedy was considered effective, rather than the ingredients used.

The connection between the remedies and the humoral theory that created them was usually hidden in private recipe collections, but one collection, British Library Manuscript Sloane 3859, offers unusual insight into the logic behind particular humoral remedies.[85] It is an anonymous recipe book, very well organized, and likely recopied as it is neat and does not look like a collection of recipes accumulated haphazardly over time. The book contains medical recipes similar to those in other collections, but it begins with a table that lists ingredients based on their humoral properties: hot and dry, cold and dry, hot and moist, cold and moist. This illustrates the link between particular remedies for reproductive disorders and their humoral causes. A common explanation for infertility was an excess of cold and moisture, and the reproductive recipes in this book usually used ingredients that the author identified as 'hot and dry', properties that were useful for countering those humoral excesses. One recipe for 'Barrennesse' suggested bruising sage and infusing it in a gallon of milk combined with sack (a form of dry wine). This infusion should be heated and combined with 'as much sugar as will make it gratefull to tast [e]'. The resulting sage 'juice' should be combined with water and drunk every morning and, if the patient desired, also every night.[86] In the table at the beginning of Sloane 3859, the author listed sage as having 'hot and dry' properties.[87] It was also used in recipes for curing colds and other similarly cold and moist conditions.[88] None of the other ingredients in the recipe (milk, sack and sugar) appear in the table, which is comprised primarily of herbs, suggesting that the sage was considered the 'active ingredient' in the cure, while the other ingredients were merely a means for conveying the herb. The index at the end of the book listed various medical conditions and the herbs that may be used to treat them, another unusual feature in a manuscript recipe book. In that list, sage appeared not only under 'barrennesse to helpe' but also under 'abortion to hinder' as well as 'courses to provoke'.[89] Tansy also appeared as a remedy for amenorrhea and to prevent miscarriages, while 'clary' and mercury (a chemical rather than herbal remedy) appeared as cures for both infertility and amenorrhea. The fact that the same ingredients were used to prevent miscarriages, promote fertility and encourage menstruation suggests that women would have tried to menstruate in order to conceive rather than as a form of abortion, although the category 'courses to provoke' also included some herbs that were used as abortifacients. Reproductive recipes in other collections used many of the same ingredients listed in Sloane 3589, indicating that while most recipe collectors did not concern themselves with explanatory models for their remedies, they nonetheless worked within the humoral framework and used ingredients which were meant to correct the humoral imbalances that caused infertility or a predilection to miscarry.

While most reproductive recipes were based on humoral logic, some were distinctly not part of that system and relied on a logic that a modern interpretation would call 'magical'. Their perceived effectiveness was derived from various occult explanations such as sympathetic relations.[90] These recipes were not distinguished in the books in any significant way and were treated like the humoral recipes, suggesting that from the patient's perspective there was no particular difference between the types. Johanna St John suggested that tying a dried toad around the waist would serve to prevent miscarriages. In the European folkloric tradition, toads had a long association with fertility, in part because it was believed that the uterus resembled a toad.[91] St John also noted that a woman who needed to deliver a dead child should drink the breast milk of another woman. Presumably the milk of a woman who had already given birth would aid in the delivery of the stillborn child.[92] Aletheia Talbot Howard suggested a powder made from boar's testicles in order to cause conception, clearly a case in which the boar's reproductive organs were meant to aid in reproduction.[93] Howard may have copied that recipe from Andrew Boorde's *Breviery of Healthe* (1552).[94] There are also several recipes which called for laying various substances on the body, sometimes without directly touching the skin. One recipe attributed to the unnamed wife of Richard Napier suggested that delivery would be speeded by taking 'a handfull of inset leekes boile and lay to the navell in a close in lot as may suffered'.[95] Another recipe book suggested dipping a piece of white toast in muscadine wine and laying this on the navel.[96] In his 1656 guide to making 'simples', William Cole listed a few 'popular' beliefs regarding the medical use of plants; these included the idea that tying the seeds of a particular plant to a woman's arm could 'helpe Barrenesse'.[97] The differentiation between different kinds or types of remedies was less important to patients than their perceived efficacy. This was also true for choices made about advice from paid practitioners, with the added complication that, as noted, women were less likely to seek fertility advice from male practitioners owing to considerations of modesty as well as women's perceived expertise on reproductive matters.

Once a woman decided that the treatments available at home were insufficient for her needs, she could seek advice from paid medical practitioners, people who provided their services in the medical marketplace, advertised their expertise and knowledge in treating specific complaints, and offered a range of treatments including humoral medicine, chemical medicine, folk medicine, astrology, patent medicines, panaceas and magical cures. Some of these medical practitioners were women, such as Mary Trye, the daughter of a chemical physician and a chemical practitioner herself, who advertised her ability to treat numerous conditions, including 'diseases attending women', meaning hysterical fits, green sickness, obstructions and barrenness.[98] She identified these conditions as delicate and inappropriate for general discussion, and in doing so used the perceived expertise of women on reproductive matters in order to sell her medical services more effectively. 'The diseases incident to this sex are many,' she wrote in her advertisement 'and not proper here largely to be discoursed on; therefore I purposely omit them, and shall only say that they have effectual remedies.'[99] Another female practitioner, advertising anonymously in the Old Bailey proceedings in the early eighteenth century, described herself as a 'gentlewoman who practiced Physic in Distempers incident to her own Sex'.[100] She claimed to have recently returned to England, and wished to notify 'those Ladies who have lamented her absence' of her return. The reason for this lament was the 'poisonous Mercurials, and Bismuth Powder sold at chemists, apothecaries and powder shops, they have been forced to make use of for want of her excellent Preparations'. Now that she had returned, however, she not only advertised a variety of cosmetics, but also 'her Advice in Physic . . . to her own Sex, who thro' Modesty cannot relate their disorders to a male physician'.[101] The practitioner presented herself as an expert specifically in female medical conditions, which she could treat because they were of 'her own Sex'. Similarly, midwife and astrologer Mary Holden advertised at the end of her 1688 almanac that she had 'Excellent Remedies for all Women troubled with Vapours, Rising of the Mother, Convultion fits . . . and all other Diseases incident to my own Sex'. Her target audience was women, and she presented herself as an expert on conditions specific to women, suggesting that as a woman she was particularly suited to treat them.[102]

Female medical practitioners are most visible in the records when they were charged with unlicensed practice or otherwise came before the court. Margaret Pelling describes women who were censured for providing pregnancy testing or similar reproductive advice in London.[103] In 1597, a woman came before the court in Norfolk for practising medicine, but claimed that she only provided herbal remedies for women who had difficult labours.[104] There is also some limited evidence of 'wise women' who provided treatments for fertility problems and other reproductive matters. These likely offered a combination of herbal remedies and magical treatments.[105] One such 'wise woman' may have been Jane Hawkins, a member of Anne Hutchinson's heretical church in Massachusetts, who was accused by Hutchinson's enemies of practising medicine as a witch, and was 'wonted to give drinkes to other Women to cause them to conceive', which, according to her accusers, caused the women in question to give birth to monsters.[106] Of course magical treatments were not solely the purview of female practitioners, nor were they limited to practitioners of folk magic. Several collections written by learned magicians and alchemists in this period contained spells to cause conception or protect women during pregnancy and labour. They involved the use of alchemical sigils associated with Venus, the use of sympathetic magic and the inscription of religious words or the names of God.[107] One spell to cause conception suggested writing Psalm 33, 'Exultate iusti in domino', together with a set of occult characters and some perfumes, and 'laye them to her right arme, and she shall conceave'.[108]

Women also sold some cure-alls and patent medicines for fertility-related matters. After Nicholas Culpeper's death in 1654, his wife Alice began marketing a 'universal' cure called *Aurum Potabile* (a common alchemical preparation), which she claimed was based on her husband's recipe. The cure was advertised within printed copies of Culpeper's works and was to be 'administered by a Physitian in her [Alice Culpeper's] house neer London, on the East side of Spittle-fields, next door to the Red Lyon'. Among the *Aurum Potabile's* properties, 'It causeth Women subject to Abortion, or Miscarriage, to go their time: and yet being given when the time comes, it causeth a speedy and easie delivery', so that its ability to prevent premature labour did not interfere with its aid for timely births, and it could also be used to 'provoke the terms'.[109] Like Mary Trye and other female practitioners, Alice Culpeper relied on her family connections to a male practitioner in order to legitimize her practice. She also explicitly noted that a physician would be administering the cure, circumventing the potential legal complications of acting as an unlicensed practitioner.[110]

Like their female counterparts, male medical practitioners also advertised their services as experts on the treatment of fertility problems. In doing so, they had to overcome the potential problem of modesty as well as their perceived inexperience with the female body. Learned practitioners, such as the physician James Wolveridge, the iatrochemist Nicholas Sudell or the herbalist and astrologer Nicholas Culpeper, promoted their practices by publishing midwifery manuals, in which they highlighted the limitations of women's experiential knowledge of reproduction and the advantages of a more systematic approach to conception, pregnancy and childbirth.[111] Culpeper addressed his *Directory* to the midwives of England, claiming to provide them with the knowledge that the College of Physicians was hiding from them. While he recognized the importance of midwives, he also asked them to 'know [their] ignorance in that part of physic which is the basis of [their] act'. This ignorance, of course, Culpeper could end, by sharing the 'little sparks of knowledge' that he held on the subject. He presented himself as an expert on reproduction and childbirth (through the knowledge given to him by God), although he also recognized that midwives had experiential knowledge of reproduction and asked them to use that knowledge in order to correct any errors in the book.[112] Physician James Wolveridge's introductory material to his *Speculum Matricis*, a book filled with reproductive advice not solely focused on childbirth, similarly identified the book as bringing knowledge to women and midwives. He stated that 'women were most fit to help women in their deliveries, by reason of the modesty of their sex', but he also presented himself as having experience aiding women in childbirth. As such, his book claimed to bring medical knowledge to midwives in such a way that it would be 'suitable to the meanest capacity' and meant 'to inform the less knowing'.[113]

Midwifery manuals and other printed health guides contained some remedies for treating fertility problems, and these were similar to those that appeared in private recipe collections. Indeed, some of the recipes in private collections were directly copied from printed manuals. Remedies printed in manuals written by medical practitioners suggest some of the treatments that those practitioners would have prescribed to their patients, although they likely kept some remedies to themselves. Nicholas Sudell, for example, noted explicitly that only the most basic of his remedies appeared in his *Women's Friend*, while he would be happy to provide more advanced chemical remedies as part of his practice.[114] One of the earliest popular medical manuals in English was *The Breviary of Healthe*, written in 1552 by 'Andrew Boorde, of Phisicke Doctour, an Englishe Man'.[115] Boorde was careful to clarify that his work was not meant to supplant the work of physicians, but only to serve as an addition to it. He warned women who were concerned about miscarriages 'to beware what medicines they doo take except it be of by the councel of expert doctours of physicke'.[116] He nevertheless suggested several remedies to aid in this matter, including St John's wort, anise and fennel.[117] While this medicine came from the arsenal of herbal remedies, Boorde's cure for barren women was based on sympathetic magic. He suggested that 'baren women use to eat en pouder [in powdered form] the matrix [womb] of an hare or drynke the pouder of the stones of a bore with wyne'.[118] Rabbits and hares were considered useful for fertility because of their notoriously high rate of reproduction. It is also obvious why both the testicles and the uterus of fertile animals were considered particularly powerful when it came to reproduction. The early midwifery manual *The Byrth of Mankinde* also suggested several remedies to aid with conception, including 'a suppository made of hare's dung and honey'.[119] Again, using material from the hare drew on its reproductive powers, while honey was a frequent ingredient in medical recipes.

While some practitioners advertised their practices indirectly through medical manuals, there were also explicit advertisements for medical services. Often these advertised specific patent medicines or cure-alls, which were meant to treat a range of illnesses. Infertility was frequently listed among the conditions that such panaceas treated. The medical empiric William Salmon, who also practised chemical and astrological medicine, used the first pages of his 1696 household medical guide to advertise 'The Virtues and Uses of the True *Balsam de Chili*, to be had at Dr. Salmon's House, at the Blew Ball by the Ditch side, near Holborn-bridge, London'.[120] This balsam was, of course, 'excelling all others' and 'curing many inveterate, and supposed incurable Diseases'. It was described as useful for a great many conditions, including aches, pains, ulcers, gout and sciatica. However, like many other such cure-alls, it also promoted 'conception, and causes speedy and easie delivery to Women in Travel, taking away and preventing Afterpains'.[121] Another medical practitioner operating in 1700, one 'W. Elmy, Professor of Physic and Operator', placed several advertisements in the proceedings of the Old Bailey for his patent cures.[122] These included some 'Anti-Hectic Lozenges, of a very pleasant Taste, and never made publick until now, being the Prescription of a very Eminent and Ancient Physician lately Deceased', which prevented consumption, aided those suffering from heartburn, offered a cure for stones and in addition to all this 'are one of the best Medicines in the World to prevent Miscarriage'.[123]

Medical practitioners of all sorts offered treatments for fertility problems, but learned male practitioners were almost exclusive in keeping detailed records of the treatment they provided. The men who kept these records were either university-trained physicians, or learned practitioners of astrological or chemical medicine. The records reveal that they did not frequently treat women for fertility problems, doing so only in specific cases.[124] When they did offer fertility treatments, they were contacted by women directly, or sometimes by their husbands. Although their expertise was respected, the advice they gave was not always taken at face value. Patients took the advice they received and considered how best to apply it and how to integrate it with their own medical knowledge and their own understandings of their body.[125] Many of the treatments on offer were herbal remedies similar to those that circulated in private recipe collections, although some required more specialized equipment or involved more unusual methods of application, which may perhaps be attributed to their more 'professional' nature. Casebooks were also somewhat more likely to include explanations of the causes of the problem and advice to change certain lifestyle factors, which did not usually appear in private remedy collections.

In the latter half of the sixteenth century, Cambridge-educated physician Hugo Glyn kept a book of medical recipes in which he also noted treatments he had prescribed to patients.[126] Among the treatments Glyn collected were several recipes to provoke menstruation, one 'In sterilitatem', one recipe for 'the paralysis of the penis', a few recipes to facilitate conception and several recipes for aphrodisiacs, including one 'ut mulier placate viro' ('that a woman may satisfy her husband').[127] Many of these recipes appear out of context, with no association to a particular patient, but several of them are specifically associated with a Lady Talbot, who seemed to have suffered from problems with her menstruation.[128] One recipe to aid conception appeared with the note 'Gabrial Gestwycke', but it is unclear if this was the source of the recipe or the patient to whom Glyn prescribed it.[129] Some of the physician's advice had to do with lifestyle factors. For problems with sexual performance he recommended moderation in food, drink and emotion. 'Avoid anger . . . be joyful and hope for the best and be cheerful', he advised, an echo of the admonition that negative emotions could hinder conception.[130] The majority of the prescriptions were herbal remedies. At first glance they appear very similar to those collected in private recipe collections, with cinnamon, betony, roses and ginger all appearing in several of the recipes.[131] One prescription for a suppository to promote conception was based on the blood of a hare, making use of the sympathetic connection between hares and fertility. Unlike most private recipe collections, however, Glyn's recipes were written in Latin, the language of educated physicians rather than private collectors.[132] Moreover, several of the remedies were intended for direct application to the genitals. This method very rarely appeared in private collections and was more common in general medical treatises, although Jennifer Evans suggests that this was particularly true for aromatics, as smells were a more indirect way of applying treatment to the womb.[133] Among Glyn's medicines that were meant for direct application on the body was an ointment made from cherry leaves, castor oil and wax, 'in order to facilitate conception'. This was to be applied to the genitals of both the woman and the man, as was another similar recipe. Cherry leaves are not particularly aromatic, so the intention was likely not to arouse the womb through smell, but rather through some action of the ointment. Indeed, the use of wax and oil suggests something in the nature of a lubricant, as does the application to both husband and wife, although the recipe does not specify that it should be used directly before intercourse.[134] No doubt the medicine was not meant to be applied by the physician but by the patients, but the presence of recipes involving the genitals so directly is perhaps indicative of the more 'professional' aspects of treatment by a physician.

Another matter that differentiated the fertility treatments offered by some physicians from the remedies used at home or from patent medicines was the consideration given to the specific patient and the particular balance of her humours in treatment. In the mid-seventeenth century, Physician John Symcotts wrote a letter to a patient who suffered from frequent miscarriages. She was receiving treatment from another physician, but Symcotts had known her from childhood and he suggested that the 'long experience I have had of your constitution from your childhood' enabled him to offer a more accurate opinion than her current physician.[135] He indicated that the patient's miscarriages were caused by 'the ill concoction of your stomach, perverting and depraving the good nourishment it receives and possessing it with intemperate qualities; the expulsive sends down a good proportion of it to the more remote and ignoble parts as not consistent with veins has (upon the same grounds) power enough to irritate nature to expulsion, and with that, of the grateful fruit of conception'. In order to counter this, he advised vomits and purges, and

> all this while (which will be your worst task) to drink for your ordinary beer of barley-liquorice water, which I have often known to tame the sharpest and most virulent humours that are imaginable and prevented miscarriages ever after. And when you perceive yourself to be with child and shall find any signs that threaten the loss of it, trust not to astringents, inward, outward, ointments, emplasters, bleedings etc., which cannot bear up against those sharp humours that nature of necessiry must thrust out or sink under; but presently fall to the continuation of gentle purgatives till such formidable signs do disappear[136]

Symcotts then provided the patient with recipes for all of the treatments he advised, and noted that her current physician might choose to alter them. He diagnosed the problem based on his familiarity with her temperament, and prescribed treatment based on the same.

A similar concern with a patient's particular humoral condition can be seen in the treatment given by Théodore de Mayerne, the premier physician in England in the first half of the seventeenth century, to author and woman of science Margaret Cavendish, Duchess of Newcastle.[137] In 1649 Mayerne corresponded with Margaret's husband, William Cavendish, then the Marquess of Newcastle, who was in exile in France and could not visit Mayerne directly.[138] William wrote to Mayerne in order to seek advice both for himself and for his wife, who was troubled with a condition that Mayerne diagnosed as stemming from a melancholic temperament.[139] In addition to treatment of their other medical conditions, William also consulted with Mayerne about Margaret's inability to conceive. 'Touching conception,' Mayerne wrote to Newcastle in May 1648, 'I know not if in the estate she's in you ought earnestly to desire it, It is hard to get Children with good Corage, when One is Melancholy.'[140] Writing as a father who had lost children, Mayerne continued to write that once children were brought into the world 'very often one looses them, as I have try'd to my great greefe and am sory to have had them . . . '.[141] Mayerne was concerned that given Margaret's general melancholy temperament and health problems, it might be a poor decision to have children. He was willing to suggest a treatment for Margaret's infertility, but only provided she took it after she had already been cured of her other ailments. He suggested that after Margaret had been cured of her current condition by bathing at Brouge, then 'The bathes of Burbone will not be unprofitable to hir, so that she use them to purpose [in order to conceive], with good councell.'[142] Mayerne believed that both body and mind had to be healed before one could engage in a healthy reproductive process.

Taking the Waters

Mayerne's advice that Margaret Cavendish should take the waters in order to promote conception was in line with the growing practice among elite women in the seventeenth century. Recipe books and midwifery manuals noted a range of treatments for infertility, and rarely listed water cures among them, but almost all of the evidence of women actually treating fertility problems in this period is of taking the waters. The reason for this discrepancy is that there are more abundant sources for fertility problems among royal or aristocratic women, given the high political stakes of their reproduction. Water cures were an elite practice, usually requiring a lengthy visit to a spa town such as Bath or Tunbridge Wells, and such visits often included a social element such as entertaining or travelling with companions.[143] More 'typical' women were less likely to use such cures, but they were also less likely to leave any record of their treatment of fertility problems, creating a gap between the treatments that most women were advised to use and the treatments for which there is the most detailed documentation.

The growth of English spas as elite medical locations in the seventeenth and eighteenth century was connected to their uses by royal women, often, although not exclusively, to promote conception or treat frequent reproductive disorders.[144] As a result water cures gained a reputation for treating reproductive disorders that extended to popular culture as well as to medicine.[145] One poem from the 1570s about the baths at Buxton, suggested that 'The barren wife here meets her husband's love, With such success she straight doth mother prove.'[146] A later poem about Tunbridge Wells noted that the water could: 'quicken the conception'.[147] Spa towns were not always popular among upper-class women. Immediately after the Reformation, water cures actually fell out of favour, because they were associated with specific saints and with Catholic ritual.[148] However, starting in the 1570s physicians working in or near English spa towns began publishing treatises advertising the uses of their local waters, extolling the virtues of various spas and watering places, now no longer using the religious terminology of saintly cures but the medical terminology of balancing the humours.[149] These publications rehabilitated some ancient spas, chief among them Bath. In addition they promoted newly discovered waters, such as those at Tunbridge Wells, thus offering additional bathing locations that were free of any 'papist' associations.

In the process, water cures were recast in medical terminology instead of a religious one, but they did not become 'secular'. Rather, they were understood within a religious framework that saw the spas as God's particular divine gift to England and would work, like all medicine, through God's will.[150] John Jones, for example, wrote in his guide to the baths of Buxton in 1572 that patients should not despair if they were not immediately cured of their condition, but should rather pray more emphatically to God for their cure.[151] He then provided a recommended regimen for treatment that included information on the best times to bathe, how to eat, sleep and exercise while taking the waters, and also the admonition to say 'the praier in the later end of this booke, on your knees, either in the appointed places, or in your chamber, or on the Bathes' as part of the process.[152] In the prayer the supplicant acknowledged that 'the breach of they most holly lawes, which we have, to often done, is the very cause, that we be so vered, greved, diseased, and enfeabled, as a iust crosse, for our misdeeds', but asked God to cure his or her condition regardless. The physician, meanwhile, was described as 'nature's assistant', who cures patients through God's will.[153]

The decision to take the waters might come from an interaction between a patient and a physician. As noted, Théodore Mayerne advised Margaret Cavendish to take the waters for her infertility. Hans Sloane, the most prominent English physician of the late seventeenth and early eighteenth centuries, also prescribed water treatments for patients suffering from miscarriages and other reproductive ailments.[154] Although physicians prescribed water cures and advised on their proper uses, patients could also choose to take the waters without prescription, especially if they were already experienced in the use of such cures. Princess Anne initially went to Tunbridge Wells for her reproductive disorders following the advice of her physician, John Radcliffe, but she later decided to resume treatment without awaiting her physician's advice, using her past experience as a guide.[155] A frequent trope in advertisements of spas was that of patients trying them when all other treatments had failed, making water cures another available option that patients could choose, without necessarily requiring a medical practitioner to guide them.[156] Mary Whitelocke noted 'taking the waters' as a practice separate from 'physic', suggesting that early modern patients also saw this as another kind of treatment, not quite in the same category as using remedies or prescriptions. As one more competing option within the medical marketplace, spas were advertised quite aggressively by the medical practitioners who were in charge of them.

Advertisements on the virtues of medical bathing utilized much of the same language that appeared in other advertisements of cure-alls, meaning that they considered bathing a panacea that could cure almost all conditions. Like advertisements for cure-alls, pamphlets about the baths often listed reproductive matters explicitly among the problems they could cure. Unlike many purveyors of cure-alls, however, physicians who wrote advertisements for medicinal bathing sought to place water cures clearly within the framework of humoral medicine. They argued that the waters worked by altering the body's temperament or encouraging a purging or balancing of the humours. In the middle ages medical spas tended to be associated with a particular saint, and bathing was a religious ritual that was intended to bring forth saintly intercession on behalf of the patient. The baths at Buxton, for example, were associated with St Anne, patron saint of barren women, and so bathing there was meant to cure infertility.[157] After the Reformation, most baths lost their association with the saints, and their efficacy was also not seen as derived from occult means, as was the case with magical cures. In John Jones's pamphlet on those same baths at Buxton he explained that the baths cured 'Women that by reason of overmuch moisture, or contrary distemperature, be unapt to conceave. Also one such as have their whites too abundant, and that bee over watry.' The baths at Buxton also helped 'Weake men that bee unfrutefull'.[158] Jones explained that the baths could moderate the excess of moisture that was often seen as the cause of infertility, placing bathing as a practice firmly within the humoral tradition.

Some advertisements did not simply discuss the general 'properties' of the waters, but rather gave particular case studies or examples of cures. The subjects of these cures were usually described as 'gentlemen', 'gentlewomen' and 'ladies', a further indication that the baths were associated with a particular social class. Michael Stanhope's 1632 publication on the virtues of the waters near Knaresborough, Yorkshire, contained the story of Lady Hoyle, the wife of the Mayor of York, who became afflicted with a strange illness. Whenever Lady Hoyle conceived, her face began to swell and grow 'many knobs', and soon afterwards she miscarried, a problem that recurred several times. After trying every form of medicine that money could buy, she finally went to the spa for a three-week stay. Not only did her condition improve immediately, but within two months of her return home, Lady Hoyle conceived and went through a successful pregnancy, without any of her former symptoms.[159] Another example comes from the register of the cures that took place at Bath, which was published in 1685. The register described a thirty-two-year-old gentlewoman who had been married for twelve years yet failed to conceive. She became afflicted with palsy and, as in the previous example, tried every remedy possible before travelling to Bath in 1664. Following her visit she was not only cured of the palsy, but conceived. These conceptions first resulted in several miscarriages, but the story ended with a note stating that 'Dr *Carie* of *Bath* hath testified this . . . who saw the party twenty one *years* after her using the *Bath* free from the *palsey* with a numerous issue.'[160] Such case studies were meant to prove the true efficacy of the baths. Like stories of miraculous healing in the Catholic tradition, the stories follow a particular model, in which the patients suffered from a completely incurable condition which could not be solved by any treatment until she took the waters and was quickly cured.

Pamphlets notwithstanding, the best advertisement for water cures as a treatment for infertility was the use of the spas by England's queens. Henrietta-Maria, wife of Charles I, took the waters for her fertility at Wellingborough and at Tunbridge Wells in 1627, 1628 and 1629. Alvise Contarini, the Venetian ambassador to England, reported several times that Henrietta was taking the waters in order to conceive of a child. On 23 July 1627 he reported that 'The queen has gone to Wellingborough [in Northamptonshire], 150 miles away to drink some mineral waters which facilitate generation, as with no signs of anything in more than two years people naturally begin to comment on the matter.'[161] On 27 August of the same year Contarini noted that 'the king has written to his wife, who is at the baths',[162] while on 22 August 1628 the ambassador wrote that 'The king remains hunting, 50 miles away, and the queen is drinking mineral waters to facilitate child bearing, which is desirable and necessary.'[163] Henrietta Maria would eventually give birth to seven living children, but her first pregnancy in 1629 ended in a stillbirth, which she mentioned in her correspondence as a 'misfortune' or 'accident'.[164] Her first viable child was the future Charles II, born in 1630, five years after her marriage. The treatments were thus necessary while she thought she was infertile.

Henrietta-Maria's daughter in law, Catherine of Braganza, was not so fortunate in her reproduction. Catherine and Charles II were married in 1662, and when Catherine did not conceive during the first few months of the marriage, rumours began to circulate that she was barren.[165] These rumours were aided by the fact that Charles had fathered several illegitimate children by his mistresses, so that the king's fertility was well established. In July 1663, after trying medical cures for her infertility as well as the use of various holy relics which were available to her as a Catholic, Catherine travelled to Tunbridge Wells in the hopes of curing her infertility, and in the following years she returned periodically to Tunbridge or Bath for the same reason. Although Catherine conceived several times, all of these pregnancies ended in miscarriage and she never gave birth to an heir.[166]

The most famous royal visit to the baths was that of Mary of Modena, wife of James II. As noted, Mary's claim that she gave birth to a son in 1688 was the subject of much contention, and many attempts were made either to prove or disprove it. An important part of the story of the birth of the Prince of Wales was the fact that Mary had gone to Bath because she had suffered from previous miscarriages and gave birth to sickly children who did not survive, and she wanted to ensure a successful conception and a healthy pregnancy. Mary's enemies claimed that she was physically unable to keep a pregnancy to full term or give birth to viable offspring, and therefore could not have given birth to the prince.[167] When one of Mary's ladies-in-waiting, Margaret Dawson, was questioned about the queen's pregnancy, she wrote in her deposition that 'the reason of the Queens being delivered of the prince of Wailes sooner than was expected was because the bath had mayd some alteration in the Queens breeding which was that nature proved one month after she had conceived with chylde, which it had never dun before of all her children . . . '.[168] Dawson's deposition did not contradict the claim that the queen had previously miscarried and may have even been unable to have children in the past. Rather, she claimed that the bath had caused a change in the queen's 'breeding', utilizing the idea that the baths could cure certain 'distempers' and thus turn a previously infertile woman into a fertile one. James and Mary attributed the pregnancy to the visit to Bath, and after Mary conceived, the Earl of Melfort, James's Secretary of State, commissioned a marble cross to decorate the Cross Bath where Mary had bathed, a decoration which was later destroyed because it was too 'papist'.[169]

When queens went to visit the baths they were always accompanied by their ladies and other courtiers, and royal visits served not only to further the fame of the baths as medical locations but also to increase their status as social locations. Count Terriesi, the Duke of Tuscany's envoy to England, described Mary of Modena's routine while at Bath in a letter in September 1687:

> They who come from those baths say that Her Majesty is taking them very conscientiously, and has the company of other ladies, who bathe with her, the music of the Italians which constantly diverts her, and the sight of all the people who crowd around to pay their court, or to witness a hitherto unseen spectacle. In the afternoon Her Majesty drives through the valleys to the sound of the warlike instruments of the band of her Guards, and of an evening until supper-time she gives audience to all who desire it, who are not a few, the greater part of the gentry of the town and neighbourhood desiring the honour of kissing Her Majesty's hand.[170]

For aristocratic women, baths were the treatment of choice starting from the middle of the seventeenth century. Such women had their own recipe collections and also consulted with physicians and other practitioners, but bathing was often incorporated into their treatment. It is quite likely that the attraction of the baths for them was not simply their potential for a cure but also the social benefits. Taking the waters allowed royal and aristocratic women to remove themselves from certain duties, while still enjoying the company of many of their friends or courtiers. Moreover, as bathing became more popular, spa towns began developing housing and amenities for entertaining such upper-class guests, so that taking the waters was increasingly a source of pleasure as well as medicinal aid. No doubt the relatively relaxed atmosphere at the spas would have been particularly pleasant for royal women, on whom the pressures of reproduction were particularly high.

Conclusion

Decisions about how to treat fertility problems were made by patients, usually by women themselves and occasionally by their husbands. They had a wide range of options, from basic herbal remedies involving common household ingredients to a lengthy and expensive visit to a spa. What they ultimately chose likely depended on their wealth, status and the longevity and severity of their medical condition. Fertility treatments taken by ordinary women who did not conceive quickly after marriage left no real record, except as notes in private recipe books, in which there is little information about who used the recipe and for what purpose. When the stakes of reproduction were higher, as in the case of royal women, or when no child was born for many years after a marriage, more wide-ranging treatment might be sought, including consultations with physicians and the use of elaborate chemical treatments or perhaps even astrological and magical cures. Patients were agents in their own treatment, making choices about which practitioner to consult and how to use their advice. They often preferred a form of treatment that was based on taking remedies or going for a pleasant vacation at a spa, rather than more holistic changes to their lifestyle that might be advised by their physicians.

All of these medical options, however, functioned as part of a broader understanding of infertility as a condition that was part of God's plan, and that would be cured only if it was His will to do so. For many patients, prayer was the primary action to take when faced with infertility, with physic acting only as a secondary factor. Furthermore, treatment itself was accompanied by prayer, which was integrated into the process of healing. Indeed, in Whitelocke's religious narrative, it was only after she had decided to cease treatment of all kinds, and to pray more for acceptance of her barrenness than for its cure, that she conceived for the first time. This conception ended in a miscarriage, but Whitelocke nonetheless chose to interpret it as a sign that only acceptance of God's will might result in the child she desired.[171]

Notes

1. Mary Whitelocke, *Advice for Her Son Samuel*, Princeton University RTC01 Ms. 226, unnumbered.
2. Mary Fissell, 'The Politics of Reproduction in the English Reformation', *Representations* 87, no. 1 (2004): 43–81.
3. Whitelocke, *Advice for Her Son Samuel.*
4. Alexandra Walsham, *Providence in Early Modern England* (Oxford; New York: Oxford University Press, 1999). Helen Berry and Elizabeth A. Foyster, 'Childless Men in Early Modern England,' in *The Family in Early Modern England*, ed. Helen Berry and Elizabeth A. Foyster (Cambridge: Cambridge University Press, 2007), pp. 165–166. Susan Dwyer Amussen, *An Ordered Society: Gender and Class in Early Modern England* (New York: Blackwell, 1988).
5. James Joseph Bono, *The Word of God and the Languages of Man: Interpreting Nature in Early Modern Science and Medicine* (Madison: University of Wisconsin Press, 1995).
6. John Jones, *The Benefit of the Auncient Bathes of Buckstones* (Derby at the Kings Mede, 1572), p. 21.
7. Ian Mortimer, *The Dying and the Doctors: The Medical Revolution in Seventeenth-Century England* (Woodbridge: Boydell & Brewer, 2015), p. 2.
8. Daphna Oren-Magidor, 'Literate Laywomen, Male Medical Practitioners and the Treatment of Fertility Problems in Early Modern England', *Social History of Medicine* 29, no. 2 (2016): 290–310.
9. Patricia Crawford, *Women and Religion in England 1500–1720* (New York: Routledge, 1993), pp. 82–83, 209.
10. Lisa W. Smith, 'La Raillerie Des Femmes? Les Femmes, La Stérilité Et La Société En France a L'époque Moderne', in *Femmes En Fleurs, Femmes En Corps: Sang, Santé, Sexualités Du Moyen Age Aux Lumières*, ed. Cathy McClive and Nicole Pellegrin (Saint-Étienne: Publications de l'Université de Saint-Étienne, 2010), pp. 203–220.
11. For example: Christopher Haigh, 'The Continuity of Catholicism in the English Reformation', *Past & Present* 93 (1981): 37–69.
12. Mary Fissell, 'The Politics of Reproduction in the English Reformation', *Representations* 87, no. 1 (2004): 43–81.
13. Tessa Watt, *Cheap Print and Popular Piety 1550–1640* (Cambridge: Cambridge University Press, 1991), p. 327.
14. Daphna Oren-Magidor, 'From Anne to Hannah: Religious Views of Infertility in Post-Reformation England', *Journal of Women's History* 27, no. 3 (2015), 86–108.
15. Keith Thomas, *Religion and the Decline of Magic* (New York: Scribner, 1971), p. 29.

16. Susan Signe Morrison, *Women Pilgrims in Late Medieval England: Private Piety and Public Performance* (London: Routledge, 2000), p. 28. Claire M. Waters, 'Power and Authority', in *A Companion to Middle English Hagiography*, ed. Sarah Salih (Woodbridge; Rochester, NY: D.S. Brewer, 2006), p. 84.
17. Morrison, *Women Pilgrims in Late Medieval England*, p. 24.
18. Gail McMurray Gibson, 'Saint Anne and the Religion of Childbed: Some East Anglian Texts and Talismans', in *Interpreting Cultural Symbols: Saint Anne in Late Medieval Society*, ed. Kathleen M. Ashley and Pamela Sheingorn (Athens: University of Georgia Press, 1990), pp. 106–107.
19. Ronald C. Finucane, *Miracles and Pilgrims: Popular Beliefs in Medieval England* (Totowa, NJ: Rowman and Littlefield, 1977), p. 105.
20. James Craigie Robertson, *Materials for the History of Thomas Becket, Archbishop of Canterbury* (London: Longman, 1875), pp. 264–265.
21. Diana Webb, *Pilgrimage in Medieval England* (London: Hambledon and London, 2000), pp. 140, 97–98. John Blair, *St Frideswide's Monastery at Oxford: Archaeological and Architectural Studies* (Gloucester: Alan Sutton, 1990), pp. 274–275.
22. Thomas, *Religion and the Decline of Magic*, p. 32.
23. Thomas, *Religion and the Decline of Magic*, p. 40. L. B. Pinto, 'The Folk Practice of Gynecology and Obstetrics in the Middle Ages', *Bulletin of the History of Medicine* 47, no. 5 (1973): 513.
24. Finucane, *Miracles and Pilgrims: Popular Beliefs in Medieval England*, pp. 67–70. Henry Mayr-Harting, 'Functions of a Twelfth-Century Shrine: The Miracles of St Frideswide', in *Studies in Medieval History Presented to R.H.C. Davis*, ed. Henry Mayr-Harting and R.I. Moore (London: Hambledon Press, 1985), p. 196.
25. James Rattue, *The Living Stream: Holy Wells in Historical Context* (Woodbridge: Boydell Press, 1995), p. 55.
26. Blair, *St Frideswide's Monastery at Oxford*, pp. 274–275.
27. William Fleetwood, *The Life and Miracles of St. Wenefride* (London: Printed for S. Buckley, 1713), p. 109.
28. Alexandra Walsham, 'Holywell, Contesting Sacred Space in Post-Reformation Wales', in *Sacred Space in Early Modern Europe*, ed. Will Coster and Andrew Spicer (Cambridge: Cambridge University Press, 2005), p. 230.
29. *An Account of the Reasons of the Nobility and Gentry's Invitation of His Highness the Prince of Orange into England* (London: Printed for Nathanael Ranew, and Jonathan Robinson, 1688), p. 23.
30. Fissell, 'The Politics of Reproduction in the English Reformation', 67.
31. Jacques Gélis, *History of Childbirth: Fertility, Pregnancy and Birth in Early Modern Europe* (Boston, MA: Rosemary Morris, 1991), p. 17.

32. Mary Fissell, *Vernacular Bodies: The Politics of Reproduction in Early Modern England* (Oxford: Oxford University Press, 2004), p. 231.
33. Frances Elizabeth Dolan, *Whores of Babylon: Catholicism, Gender, and Seventeenth-Century Print Culture* (Ithaca, NY: Cornell University Press, 1999), p. 153. The prohibition against a Catholic monarch in England still stands, but the prohibition on a Catholic consort was cancelled in the Succession to the Crown Act of 2013.
34. Fissell, 'The Politics of Reproduction in the English Reformation', 44.
35. Gélis, *History of Childbirth*, p. 92.
36. John Bale, *The Actes of Englysh Votaryes Comprehendynge Their Vnchast Practyses* (Antwerp: By S. Mierdman, 1546), frontispiece.
37. Bale, *The Actes of Englysh Votaryes*, p. 32.
38. Jean Barrin, *The Monk Unvail'd: Or, a Facetious Dialogue, Discovering the Several Intrigues, and Subtil Practises, Together with the Lewd and Scandalous Lives of Monks, Fryers, and Other Pretended Religious Votaries of the Church of Rome* (London: Printed for Jonathan Edwin, 1678), p. 80.
39. Alexandra Walsham, *Providence in Early Modern England* (Oxford: Oxford University Press, 1999). Tessa Watt, *Cheap Print and Popular Piety, 1550–1640* (Cambridge: Cambridge University Press, 1991). David Cressy, *Bonfires & Bells: National Memory and the Protestant Calendar in Elizabethan and Stuart England* (Berkeley: University of California Press, 1989).
40. Walsham, *Providence in Early Modern England*, p. 12.
41. Thomas, *Religion and the Decline of Magic*, p. 136.
42. Oren-Magidor, 'From Anne to Hannah: Religious Views of Infertility in Post-Reformation England'.
43. Thomas Bentley, *The Monument of Matrones: Conteining Seuen Seuerall Lamps of Virginitie* (London: H. Denham, 1582), pp. 6–7.
44. Bentley, *The Monument of Matrones*, table of contents.
45. Vivienne Larminie, 'Hieron, Samuel (Bap. 1572, D. 1617)', in *Oxford Dictionary of National Biography, Online ed.*, ed. Lawrence Goldman (Oxford: Oxford University Press, 2004).
46. Samuel Hieron, *A Helpe Vnto Deuotion* (London: Printed by H. Lownes for Samuell Macham, 1611), p. 156.
47. Hieron, *A Helpe Vnto Deuotion*, p. 156.
48. Hieron, *A Helpe Vnto Deuotion*, pp. 157–159.
49. Cotton Mather, *Ornaments for the Daughters of Zion, or, the Character and Happiness of a Vertuous Woman* (Cambridge, MA: Printed by S.G. and B.G. for Samuel Phillips, 1692), pp. 88–89.
50. Mather, *Ornaments for the Daughters of Zion*, pp. 88–89.
51. Oren-Magidor, 'From Anne to Hannah: Religious Views of Infertility in Post-Reformation England'.

52. Doreen Evenden, *Popular Medicine in Seventeenth-Century England* (Bowling Green, OH: Bowling Green State University Popular Press, 1988). Harold John Cook, *The Decline of the Old Medical Regime in Stuart London* (Ithaca, NY: Cornell University Press, 1986). Andrew Wear, *Knowledge and Practice in English Medicine, 1550–1680* (Cambridge: Cambridge University Press, 2000).
53. Elaine Leong and Sara Pennell, 'Recipe Collections and the Currency of Medical Knowledge in the Early Modern "Medical Marketplace"', in *Medicine and the Market in England and Its Colonies, c.1450–c.1850*, ed. Mark S.R. Jenner and Patrick Wallis (Basingstoke: Palgrave Macmillan, 2007), p. 134. Elaine Leong, 'Making Medicines in the Early Modern Household', *Bulletin of the History of Medicine* 82, no. 1 (2008): 147. Andrew Wear, 'Religious Beliefs and Medicine in Early Modern England', in *Health and Healing in Early Modern England: Studies in Social and Intellectual History*, ed. Andrew Wear (Aldershot: Ashgate, 1998), p. 145. Cook, *The Decline of the Old Medical Regime in Stuart London*, p. 30.
54. Daphna Oren-Magidor, 'Literate Laywomen, Male Medical Practitioners and the Treatment of Fertility Problems in Early Modern England'.
55. Alisha Rankin, 'Duchess, Heal Thyself: Elisabeth of Rochlitz and the Patient's Perspective in Early Modern Germany', *Bulletin of the History of Medicine* 82, no. 1 (2008): 109–144. Roy Porter, 'The Patient's View', *Theory and Society* 14 (1985): 175–198. Leigh Whaley, *Women and the Practice of Medical Care in Early Modern Europe, 1400–1800* (Basingstoke: Palgrave Macmillan, 2011), p. 137.
56. The same situation, in which women were blamed and treated for fertility problems despite a theoretical recognition that men could be sterile, also occurred in France, as shown in Lisa W. Smith, 'La Raillerie Des Femmes? Les Femmes, La Stérilité Et La Société En France a L'époque Moderne', in *Femmes En Fleurs, Femmes En Corps: Sang, Santé, Sexualités Du Moyen Age Aux Lumières*, ed. Cathy McClive and Nicole Pellegrin (Saint-Étienne: Publications de l'Université de Saint-Étienne, 2010), pp. 203–220.
57. Jennifer Evans, '"They Are Called Imperfect Men": Male Infertility and Sexual Health in Early Modern England', *Social History of Medicine* 29, no. 2 (2014): 311–332.
58. Berry and Foyster, 'Childless Men in Early Modern England'. Samuel Pepys, *The Diary of Samuel Pepys*, vol. 5 (London: Harper Collins, 2000), p. 124.
59. Pepys, *The Diary of Samuel Pepys*, p. 124.
60. Pepys, *The Diary of Samuel Pepys.*
61. Pepys was obsessed with matters of health, but rarely recorded consulting physicians: Porter, 'The Patient's View'.

62. Oren-Magidor, 'Literate Laywomen, Male Medical Practitioners and the Treatment of Fertility Problems in Early Modern England'.
63. Oren-Magidor, 'Literate Laywomen, Male Medical Practitioners and the Treatment of Fertility Problems in Early Modern England'.
64. Jayne Elisabeth Archer, 'Women and Chymistry in Early Modern England: The Manuscript Receipt Book (c. 1616) of Sarah Wigges', in *Gender and Scientific Discourse in Early Modern Culture*, ed. Kathleen P. Long (Farnham: Ashgate, 2010). On medical professionalism in this period, see: Harold John Cook, 'Good Advice and Little Medicine: The Professional Authority of Early Modern English Physicians', *Journal of British Studies* 33, no. 1 (1994): 1–31.
65. Wear, *Knowledge and Practice in English Medicine, 1550–1680*, p. 22. Thomas, *Religion and the Decline of Magic*, p. 223. Karen O'Brien, *White Magic and the Cunning Folk: Charms and Blessings in Northwest England* (Liverpool: Bluecoat Press, 2001), p. 28. *Book of Magic and Charms*, Bodl. MS. e. Museo 243, f. 13.
66. Nicholas Culpeper, *A Directory for Midwives: Or, a Guide for Women, in Their Conception, Bearing, and Suckling Their Children* (London: Printed by Peter Cole, 1651), p. 137.
67. Leong, 'Making Medicines in the Early Modern Household', 147. Cook, *The Decline of the Old Medical Regime in Stuart London*, p. 48. Whaley, *Women and the Practice of Medical Care in Early Modern Europe, 1400–1800*, pp. 131–149.
68. Leong and Pennell, 'Recipe Collections and the Currency of Medical Knowledge in the Early Modern "Medical Marketplace"'.
69. Rankin, 'Duchess, Heal Thyself' has suggested that this made remedies more attractive than a full treatment regimen, because they did not require a complete change in lifestyle.
70. See for example David Cressy, *Birth, Marriage, and Death: Ritual, Religion, and the Life-Cycle in Tudor and Stuart England* (Oxford: Oxford University Press, 1997), pp. 49–50.
71. *Seventeenth-Century English Recipe Books: Cooking, Physic and Chirurgery in the Works of Elizabeth Talbot Grey and Aletheia Talbot Howard* (Aldershot: Ashgate, 2008), p. 194.
72. Jennifer Evans, '"Gentle Purges Corrected with Hot Spices, Whether They Work or Not, Do Vehemently Provoke Venery": Menstrual Provocation and Procreation in Early Modern England', *Social History of Medicine* 25, no. 1 (2011): 2–19. Lisa W. Smith, 'Imagining Women's Fertility before Technology', *Journal of Medical Humanities* 31, no. 1 (2010): 69–79.
73. Elaine Leong, '"Herbals She Peruseth": Reading Medicine in Early Modern England', *Renaissance Studies* 28, no. 4 (2014): 556–578.

74. Leong, '"Herbals She Peruseth": Reading Medicine in Early Modern England'. Wear, *Knowledge and Practice in English Medicine, 1550–1680*, p. 42.
75. Rankin, 'Duchess, Heal Thyself: Elisabeth of Rochlitz and the Patient's Perspective in Early Modern Germany', 112. Cook, *The Decline of the Old Medical Regime in Stuart London*, p. 28.
76. John Davall, *Medical Recipe Book* BL Sloane MS 1812, f. 39. *Medical Recipes*, Bodl. Ashmole 1489, f. 78. *Medical Recipes Attributed to Richard Napier's Wife*, BL Ashmole 1390, f. 81. *Seventeenth-Century English Recipe Books*, p. 90. Elizabeth Jacobs, *Medical Recipes*, WL MSS 3009, f. 74.
77. *Medical Recipe Book*, WL MS 7391, f. 68. Elizabeth Okover, *Medical Recipes*, WL MS 3712, f. 75.
78. Jennifer Evans, *Aphrodisiacs, Fertility and Medicine in Early Modern England* (London: Royal Historical Society, 2014), p. 95.
79. Jacobs, *Medical Recipes*, f. 76.
80. Johanna St. John, *Medical Recipes*, WL MS 4338, f. 203. Katherine Palmer, *Medical Recipes*, WL MS 7976, f. 110.
81. *Book of Medical Recipes*, FSL MS v.a. 361, f. 29.
82. *Seventeenth-Century English Recipe Books*, p. 53. *Book of Medical Recipes*, FSL MS v.a. 361, f. 29. Elizabeth Freke, *Medical Recipes*, BL Add. MSS 45718, ff. 229, 33.
83. John Davall, *Medical Recipe Book*, BL Sloane MS 1812, f. 39.
84. *Seventeenth-Century English Recipe Books*, p. 53.
85. *Medical Recipe Book,* BL Sloane MSS 3859, I have been unable to locate any additional information about this text, such as who may have compiled it.
86. BL Sloane MSS 3859, f. 23.
87. BL Sloane MSS 3859, f. 23.
88. BL Sloane MSS 3859, f. 110.
89. BL Sloane MSS 3859, ff. 110–111.
90. For more on sympathetic magic in the early modern period, see: Edward Muir, *Ritual in Early Modern Europe* (Cambridge: Cambridge University Press, 1997), pp. 46–47. Owen Davies, *Popular Magic: Cunning Folk in English History* (London: Hambledon Continuum, 2007).
91. Marija Gimbutas, *The Goddesses and Gods of Old Europe, 6500–3500 BC, Myths and Cult Images* (Berkeley: University of California, 1982), p. 175–178.
92. Johanna St John, *Medical Recipes*, ff. 42, 206.
93. *Seventeenth-Century English Recipe Books*, p. 201.
94. Andrew Boorde, *The Breuiary of Healthe, for All Maner of Sicknesses and Diseases* (London: Wyllyam Powell, 1552), p. xxxiiii.
95. *Medical Recipes Attributed to Richard Napier's Wife*, f. 81.
96. *Book of Medical Recipes*, FSL MS v.a. 361, f. 29v.

97. William Coles, *The Art of Simpling. An Introduction to the Knovvledge and Gathering of Plants.* (London: Printed by J.G. for Nathaniel Brook, 1656), p. 71.
98. Mary Trye, *Medicatrix, or, the Woman-Physician* (London: Printed by T.R. & N.T, 1675), advertisement. Oren-Magidor, 'Literate Laywomen, Male Medical Practitioners and the Treatment of Fertility Problems in Early Modern England'.
99. Trye, *Medicatrix, or, the Woman-Physician* advertisement. Oren-Magidor, 'Literate Laywomen, Male Medical Practitioners and the Treatment of Fertility Problems in Early Modern England'.
100. *Old Bailey Proceedings Advertisements, 30 June 1714.*
101. *Old Bailey Proceedings Advertisements, 30 June 1714.*
102. A.S. Weber, 'Women's Early Modern Medical Almanacs in Historical Context,' *English Literary Renaissance* 33, no. 3 (2003): 358–402. Mary Holden, *The Womens Almanack for the Year of Our Lord 1688* (London: Printed by J. Millet, 1688).
103. Margaret Pelling, *Medical Conflicts in Early Modern London: Patronage, Physicians, and Irregular Practitioners 1550–1640* (Oxford: Oxford University Press, 2003), p. 210.
104. Paul Hair, *Before the Bawdy Court: Selections from Church Court and Other Records Relating to the Correction of Moral Offences in England, Scotland and New England, 1300–1800* (London: Paul Elek, 1972), p. 41.
105. Wear, *Knowledge and Practice in English Medicine, 1550–1680*, p. 22. Thomas, *Religion and the Decline of Magic*, pp. 211–219.
106. Edward Johnson, *Johnson's Wonder-Working Providence 1628–1651* (New York: Scribner, 1910), p. 132. Carol F. Karlsen, *The Devil in the Shape of a Woman: Witchcraft in Colonial New England* (New York: Norton, 1998), p. 16. Thomas, *Religion and the Decline of Magic*, p. 223.
107. *Tract on Magic*, BL Sloane MS 3851, f. 9 v. *Book of Magic and Charms*, f. 4v. *Tractati Magici*, British Library Sloane MS 3846, f. 52.
108. *Book of Magic and Charms*, f. 13.
109. Nicholas Culpeper, *Pharmacopoeia Londinensis, or, the London Dispensatory* (London: Printed by Peter Cole, 1659), final page.
110. Jennifer Evans, '"The Doctor's Wife (by the Blessing of God) Helps Barrenness": Gender and Infertility Treatments in Early Modern England', in *Gender, Health and Medicine in Historical Perspective (Forthcoming)*, ed. Sarah Toulalan. Margaret Pelling, 'Thoroughly Resented? Older Women and the Medical Role in Early Modern London', in *Women, Science and Medicine, 1500–1700: Mothers and Sisters of the Royal Society*, ed. Lynette Hunter and Sarah Hutton (Stroud: Sutton, 1997). Pelling, *Medical Conflicts in Early Modern London.*

111. James Wolveridge, *Speculum Matricis Hybernicum, or, the Irish Midwives Handmaid* (London: Printed by E. Okes, 1670). Culpeper, *A Directory for Midwives.* Nicholas. Sudell, *Mulierum Amicus: Or, the Womans Friend* (London, 1666). Oren-Magidor, 'Literate Laywomen, Male Medical Practitioners and the Treatment of Fertility Problems in Early Modern England'. Wendy D. Churchill, *Female Patients in Early Modern Britain: Gender, Diagnosis, and Treatment* (Farnham: Ashgate, 2012). Eve Keller, 'The Subject of Touch: Medical Authority in Early Modern Midwifery', in *Sensible Flesh: On Touch in Early Modern Culture*, ed. E.D. Harvey (Philadelphia: University of Pennsylvania Press, 2003).
112. Culpeper, *A Directory for Midwives*, epistle dedicatory.
113. Wolveridge, *Speculum Matricis Hybernicum, or, the Irish Midwives Handmaid* epistle dedicatory and preface.
114. Sudell, *Mulierum Amicus: Or, the Womans Friend*, p. 5.
115. Boorde, *The Breuiary of Healthe*, frontispiece.
116. Boorde, *The Breuiary of Healthe*, p. viii.
117. Boorde, *The Breuiary of Healthe*, p. viii.
118. Boorde, *The Breuiary of Healthe*, p. xxxiii.
119. Eucharius Roeslin, *The Byrth of Mankynde, Newly Translated out of Laten into Englysshe* (London: By Thomas Raynalde, 1540), p. lxxxv.
120. William Salmon, *The Family-Dictionary, or, Household Companion* (London: Printed for H. Rhodes 1696), after preface.
121. Salmon, *The Family-Dictionary, or, Household Companion*, after preface.
122. *Old Bailey Proceedings Advertisements, August 28, 1700.*
123. *Old Bailey Proceedings Advertisements, August 28, 1700.*
124. Oren-Magidor, 'Literate Laywomen, Male Medical Practitioners and the Treatment of Fertility Problems in Early Modern England'.
125. Rankin, 'Duchess, Heal Thyself: Elisabeth of Rochlitz and the Patient's Perspective in Early Modern Germany'. Oren-Magidor, 'Literate Laywomen, Male Medical Practitioners and the Treatment of Fertility Problems in Early Modern England'.
126. Hugo Glynn, *Medicinal Recipes*, WL MSS 8541.
127. Glynn, *Medicinal Recipes*, ff. 108, 230v, 34, 35, 36. The text of Glyn's book is mostly in Latin, but there is an English translation by Lillian Gertrude Ping at the Wellcome Library). For more on aphrodisiacs, see: Evans, *Aphrodisiacs, Fertility and Medicine in Early Modern England.*
128. Glynn, *Medicinal Recipes*, f. 96v.
129. Glynn, *Medicinal Recipes*, 241.
130. Glynn, *Medicinal Recipes*, 229.
131. Glynn, *Medicinal Recipes*, 236, 31.
132. Irma Taavitsainen and Päivi Pahta, *Medical Writing in Early Modern English* (Cambridge: Cambridge University Press, 2011), pp.13–14.

133. Philip Barrough, *The Methode of Phisicke Conteyning the Causes, Signes, and Cures of Invvard Diseases in Mans Body* (Imprinted at London: By Thomas Vautroullier, 1583), p. 142. Evans, *Aphrodisiacs, Fertility and Medicine in Early Modern England*, p. 91. Jennifer Evans, 'Female Barrenness, Bodily Access and Aromatic Treatments in Seventeenth-Century England', *Historical Research* 87, no. 237 (2014): 423–443.
134. The Latin was 'pudenda et partes virium', literally 'the shameful and the man parts'. Ping translated it as 'the organs of generation', but this elides both the specificity of the text and the fact that it refers to both the man and the woman. Glynn, *Medicinal Recipes*, ff. 234, 31.
135. John Symcotts, *A Seventeenth Century Doctor and His Patients: John Symcotts, 1592–1662* (Bedford: Bedfordshire Record Society, 1951), pp. 17–18.
136. Symcotts, *A Seventeenth Century Doctor and His Patients: John Symcotts, 1592–1662*, pp. 17–18.
137. For more on Mayerne see Hugh Trevor-Roper, *Europe's Physician: The Various Life of Sir Théodore De Mayerne* (New Haven, CT: Yale University Press, 2006).On Mayerne's treatment of patients with reproductive disorders see Oren-Magidor, 'Literate Laywomen, Male Medical Practitioners and the Treatment of Fertility Problems in Early Modern England'.
138. William Cavendish, *Letter to Théodore De Mayerne, 1649*, University of Nottingham Library PW V 90/8.
139. Cavendish, *Letter to Théodore De Mayerne, 1649*, f. 20v.
140. Cavendish, *Letter to Théodore De Mayerne, 1649*, ff. 19v–20.
141. Cavendish, *Letter to Théodore De Mayerne, 1649*, ff. 19v–20.
142. Cavendish, *Letter to Théodore De Mayerne, 1649*, f. 20.
143. Peter Borsay, *The Image of Georgian Bath, 1700–2000: Towns, Heritage, and History* (Oxford: Oxford University Press, 2000). Melville, *Society at Royal Tunbridge Wells in the Eighteenth Century and After.*
144. Jean Manco, 'The Cross Bath', *Bath History* 2 (1988).
145. On royal visits to treat fertility problems at spas see: Public Record Office of Great Britain, *CSPVen*, vol. 20 (London: HMSO, 1864), p. 297. Princess Anne, *Letters to Sarah Churchill, 1685*, British Library Add. MSS 61414, f. 12. Margaret Dawson, *Deposition on the Birth of the Prince of Wales*, BL Add. MSS 26657, f. 18. Anthony Hamilton, *Memoirs of the Comte De Gramont* (London: Folio Society, 1965), p. 210.
146. Bruce Osborne and Cora Weaver, *Aquae Britannia: Rediscovering 17th Century Springs & Spas* (Malvern: Cora Weaver, 1996), p. 113.
147. *Memoranda and Poems*, British Library Sloane MS 2348, f. 24.
148. Robert Hutchinson, *Thomas Cromwell: The Rise and Fall of Henry VIII's Most Notorious Minister* (New York: Thomas Dunne Books, 2009), pp. 161–162. W.H. Robertson, *A Hand-Book to the Peak of Derbyshire,*

and to the Use of the Buxton Mineral Waters (England: Bradbury & Evans, 1854), pp. 14–15.
149. For a comprehensive survey of publications about baths in early modern England see Charles F. Mullett, *Public Baths and Health in England, 16th–18th Century* (Baltimore, MD: The Johns Hopkins Press, 1946).
150. Jones, *The Benefit of the Auncient Bathes of Buckstones*, p. 21. Walter Baley, *A Briefe Discours of Certain Bathes or Medicinall Waters in the Countie of Warwicke* (1587), 3. Samuel Derham, *Hydrologia Philosophica* (Oxford: Printed by Leon. Lichfield for John Howell, 1685), p. 33.
151. Jones, *The Benefit of the Auncient Bathes of Buckstones*, p. 5.
152. Jones, *The Benefit of the Auncient Bathes of Buckstones*, p. 13.
153. Jones, *The Benefit of the Auncient Bathes of Buckstones*, pp. 21–22.
154. Anne Hamilton, *Letter to Hans Sloane, November 6, 1708*, BL Sloane MSS 4041.
155. Anne, *Letters to Sarah Churchill*, BL Add. MS 61414, ff. 34–36.
156. Thomas Guidott, *The Register of Bath or Two Hundred Observations Containing an Account of Cures Performed and Benefit Received by the Use of the Hot Waters of Bath* (London, 1694), p. 40.
157. Hutchinson, *Thomas Cromwell: The Rise and Fall of Henry Viii's Most Notorious Minister*, pp. 161–162. Robertson, *A Hand-Book to the Peak of Derbyshire, and to the Use of the Buxton Mineral Waters*, pp. 14–15.
158. Jones, *The Benefit of the Auncient Bathes of Buckstones*, p. 4.
159. Michael. Stanhope, *Cures Vvithout Care* (London: Printed by William Iones, 1632), pp. 15–16.
160. Guidott, *The Register of Bath*, p. 40.
161. Britain, *CSPVen*, p. 297.
162. Britain, *CSPVen*, p. 342.
163. Britain, *CSPVen*, p. 342.
164. Mary Anne Everett Green, *Letters of Queen Henrietta Maria, Including Her Private Correspondence with Charles I* (London: Richard Bentley, 1857), pp. 12–13.
165. Derek A. Wilson, *All the King's Women: Love, Sex and Politics in the Life of Charles II* (London: Hutchinson, 2003), p. 195.
166. Wilson, *All the King's Women: Love, Sex and Politics in the Life of Charles II*, p. 240.
167. *Depositions Pertaining to the 'Pretended' Prince of Wales*, BL Add. MSS 33286, f. 8.
168. Dawson, *Deposition on the Birth of the Prince of Wales*, f. 18.
169. Manco, 'The Cross Bath', 63.
170. M. Haile, *Queen Mary of Modena: Her Life and Letters* (New York: Dent, 1905), p. 167.
171. Whitelocke, *Advice for Her Son Samuel.*

CHAPTER 6

Conclusion

> So god at last after 16 yeares waiting and praying he gave me hopes of a child... [God] did wonderfully preserve the child in my wombe... and god did bless so to me that I went out my full time and then god did give me you my son after a hard and sore travel and I called your name Samuell because I had begged you of the lord.[1]

This was the happy ending to Mary Whitelocke's long struggle to become a mother. She named her first-born son Samuel, like the biblical Hannah, because she saw him as a direct response to her prayers, and because she had promised him to God's service, as Hannah had done. It was easy for Whitelocke to see the hand of God in her infertility and her eventual motherhood, not only because she lived within a society that believed in providence, but because she had immediate role models for this belief in biblical stories. There was no clearer evidence that God intervened in the lives of women than the biblical stories of his intervention in the pregnancies of Sarah, Rachel and Hannah, which in turn were precursors to the greatest reproductive miracle, that of the virgin birth of Christ.

Religious beliefs informed every aspect of the experience of infertility in sixteenth- and seventeenth-century England. This was expressed most explicitly by members of the godly subculture to which Mary Whitelocke and Sarah Savage belonged, but it was not limited to them. Religion was the framework through which early modern people understood fertility problems, both in the simple sense of seeing infertility as part of God's plan and

D. Oren-Magidor, *Infertility in Early Modern England*,
Early Modern History: Society and Culture,
DOI 10.1057/978-1-137-47668-5_6

in more complex ways. Religion allowed people to explain their infertility as a trial or a punishment. It gave them guidelines on how to ask for children, encouraging prayer and supplication. It reiterated biblical stories about barren women who were given a child, thus providing hope that God would hear their prayers. It also went further. Religion underlay medical explanations of infertility, as well as spiritual ones. It was the crux on which the social stigmas against infertile couples was founded. It was also the tool that explained both how medical treatments of infertility worked (by divine favour) and why they might not work (because it was not part of the divine plan). In other words, there was no aspect of infertility that was not touched, in some way, by early modern religious beliefs.

Religion played an important role in the understanding of all forms of illness and disease in the early modern period, and it should come as no surprise that it was also used to explain and treat fertility problems. However, because infertility is embedded in the broader social issues of reproduction, inheritance and gender relations it particularly highlights the religious and cultural dimensions of what might be seen as merely a medical problem. The influence of religion on perceptions of infertility were not limited to women, although the nature of early modern women's piety made them more direct in their personal spiritual ruminations about infertility. Still, male religious authors and devout female patients alike explained infertility as a test from God or a punishment of sins, and medical literature embraced this explanation, albeit implicitly, by explaining infertility as something caused by behaviours which were sinful and improper for good Christian men and women. Negative social views of infertile women and men picked up on these ideas, tying together gendered expectations regarding how manly men and womanly women should behave in relation to medical views about reproduction and with the religious perception of infertile people as potential sinners. Furthermore, while medicine and religion acted in unison to frame infertility as a fundamental problem, they also worked together to offer solutions for infertile couples, by suggesting that prayer and faith could ultimately lead either to the desired child or to an acceptance of their childlessness.

Religion framed one side of the experience of infertility, while gender relations and gender identity framed the other. In a social order that saw the family as its basic unit, failure to produce a 'proper' family, one that included children, was a problem. While many men and women in early modern England never married, let alone had children within marriage, the social norm and expectation was for men to marry women and become fathers and heads of households, and for women to express their femininity by becoming dutiful wives and mothers. Like unwed mothers and unruly women, infertility also created a sense of social unease about gender relations, highlighted in the negative stigmas associated with being infertile. These were expressed in ways that did not highlight fears over demographics or a view that hyper-fertility was positive, but rather concerns about the unruliness of women who could not produce children, and the loss of control of men who could not do their duty and provide children for their wives.

Beyond these social dimensions, however, gender played a more personal role in the lives of infertile people. For men, childlessness was a problem primarily when it was related to inheritance and to the survival of their family name. They might also desire children for personal reasons, and could certainly be loving fathers, but their view of fatherhood was seen first and foremost through their social duties. For women, the desire for children was more intimate and more closely tied to their self-identity. Bulstrode Whitelocke described Samuel's birth in his own diary, noting that Samuel was 'a childe of prayers, & whom God gave unto his Mother after she had bin 14 years marryed to her former husband, w[i]thout any childe borne'.[2] Like Mary, Bulstrode also noted God's role in this birth, but he saw it as a miracle that God did for Mary. Although Bulstrode appears to have been a devoted father to Samuel and to the other children he had with Mary, he did not *need* those children in the same way that Mary did, having already proven his virility and provided heirs for his estate before their marriage.

Moreover, infertility was more often seen as a woman's 'fault', even when there was evidence to the contrary. Although Samuel was conceived not long after Mary and Bulstrode's marriage, nowhere in Whitelocke's account of her life did she allow for the possibility that it was her first husband who had been the source of their fertility problems. She never sought an interpretation of her infertility other than that she had been tested by God, given a cross to bear so that she would learn not to enjoy the pleasures of this world too much. She noted, in fact, that Rowland Wilson, her first husband, 'did never abraid me with the want of children. Nay he was so fearfull and so tender over me: least that I should greive for want of children that I never h[e]ard him so much as wish for any before me for fear of adding to my affliction.'[3] Although Wilson also desired children, and indeed needed them as he had no heirs, Whitelocke's infertility was *her* affliction, and the sorrow was *her* sorrow.

Notes

1. Mary Whitelocke, *Advice for Her Son Samuel*, Princeton University RTC01. Ms. 226, unnumbered.
2. Bulstrode Whitelock, *The Diary of Bulstrode Whitelocke 1605–1675* (Oxford: Oxford University Press, 1990), p. 268. See also Daphna Oren-Magidor, 'From Anne to Hannah: Religious Views of Infertility in Post-Reformation England', *Journal of Women's History* 27, no. 3 (2015): 86–108.
3. Whitelocke, *Advice for Her Son Samuel.*

Bibliography

Manuscripts

Book of Magic and Charms, Bodl. MS. e. Museo 243.
Book of Magical Charms, BL Sloane MS 1311.
Book of Medical Recipes, FSL MS v.a. 361.
Depositions Pertaining to the 'Pretended' Prince of Wales, BL Add. MSS 33286.
Lectures on Anatomy, WL MS MSL.5.
Libel of the Saddler's Daughter, WSRO A1/110 1608E.
Medical Recipe Book, BL Sloane MS 3859.
Medical Recipe Book, WL MS 7391.
Medical Recipes Attributed to Richard Napier's Wife, BL Ashmole 1390.
Memoranda and Poems, BL Sloane MS 2348.
Satirical Poem on the Birth of the Prince of Wales, BL Stowe MS 305.
Tract on Magic, BL Sloane MS 3851.
Tractati Magici, BL Sloane MS 3846.
Anne, Princess, *Letters to Sarah Churchill*, British Library Add. MSS 61414–61415.
Cavendish, William, *Letter to Théodore De Mayerne, 1649*, University of Nottingham Library PW V 90/8.
Cope, Elizabeth, *Letter to Rachel Fane, Countess of Bath, September 12 1651*, KHLC u269/c273/6.
Davall, John, *Medical Recipe Book*, BL Sloane MS 1812.
Dawson, Margaret, *Deposition on the Birth of the Prince of Wales*, BL Add. MSS 26657.
Elizabeth, Countess of Bridgewater, *Devotional Book*, BL Egerton MS 607.

D. Oren-Magidor, *Infertility in Early Modern England*,
Early Modern History: Society and Culture,
DOI 10.1057/978-1-137-47668-5

Forman, Simon, *Medical Treatise*, Bodl. Ashmole MSS 390.
Freke, Elizabeth, *Medical Recipes*, BL Add. MSS 45718.
Glanville, Jane, *Letters to Her Brother John Evelyn, 1650–1651*, BL Add. MSS 78305.
Glover, Mary, *Medical Recipes*, BL Add. MSS 57944.
Glynn, Hugo, *Medicinal Recipes*, WL MSS 8541.
Hamilton, Anne, *Letter to Hans Sloane, November 6, 1708*, BL Sloane MSS 4041.
Jacobs, Elizabeth, *Medical Recipes*, WL MSS 3009.
Jurin, James, *Letters to Hans Sloane*, BL Sloane MSS 4047.
Mayerne, Théodore, *Ephemerides*, BL Sloane MS 2074.
Okover, Elizabeth, *Medical Recipes*, WL MSS 3712.
Paggit, J., *Commonplace Book*, BL Harleian MS 1026.
Palmer, Katherine, *Medical Recipes*, WL MS 7976.
Ray, John, *Letter to Hans Sloane, 1697*, BL Sloane MS 4036.
Saunders, Richard, *Medical Recipes*, Bodl. Ashmole 1489.
Savage, Sarah, *Diary of Sarah Savage*, CCRO ZD BASTEN 8.
St John, Johanna, *Medical Recipes*, WL MS 4338.
Stanhope, Hannah, *Letter to Her Sister, May 13 1685*, West Yorkshire Archive SpSt/6/1/17.
Trumbull, Elizabeth, *Prayer Book*, University of Birmingham Library 555.
Trumbull, William, *Autobiography*, Library of All Souls College, Oxford MS 317.
Whitelocke, Mary, *Advice for Her Son Samuel*, Princeton University RTC01 Ms. 226.

Printed Primary Sources

An Account of the Reasons of the Nobility and Gentry's Invitation of His Highness the Prince of Orange into England. London: Printed for Nathanael Ranew, and Jonathan Robinson, 1688.
Aristoteles Master-Piece, or, the Secrets of Generation Displayed in All the Parts Thereof. London: Printed for J. How, 1684.
A Ballad, Intituled, the Old Man's Complaint Against His Wretched Son. London: Printed for F. Coles, T. Vere and J. Wright, 1663, EBBA ID: 32615, Pepys Library, Magdalene College, Cambridge, 1.541.
The Compleat Midvvife's Practice Enlarged. London: Printed for Nathaniel Brooke, 1659.
The Compleat Midwifes Practice, in the Most Weighty *and High Concernments of the Birth of Man Containing Perfect Rules for Midwifes and Nurses*. London: Printed for Nathaniel Brooke, 1656.
Damnable Practises of Three Lincolne-Shire Witches, Joane Flower, and Her Two Daughters, Margret and Phillip Flower. London: Printed by G. Eld for Iohn Barnes, 1619.

A Discourse of the Married and Single Life. Wherein, by Discouering the Misery of the One, Is Plainely Declared the Felicity of the Other. London: Imprinted for Ionas Man, 1621.

The English Midwife Enlarged. London: Printed for Thomas Sawbridge, 1682

The Lamenting Lady, Who for the Wrongs Done to Her by a Poore Woman, for Hauing Two Children at One Burthen, Was by the Hand of God Most Strangely Punished. London: for Henry Gosson, 1620. EBBA ID: 20210, Pepys Library, Magdalene College, Cambridge, 1.44–1.45.

The Mistaken Mid-Vvife, or, Mother Mid-Night Finely Brought to Bed. London: Printed for F. Coles T. Vere J. Wright and J. Clarke, 1674.

My Dog and I. London: Printed for F. Coles, T. Vere, J. Wright, and J. Clarke, 1674.

Old Bailey Proceedings Advertisements, 28 August 1700.

Old Bailey Proceedings Advertisements, 30 June 1714.

The Scolding Wives Vindication: Or, an Answer to the Cuckold's Complaint. London: Printed for P. Brooksby. J. Deacon. J. Blare. J. Back, 1683. EBBA ID 21801, Magdalene College Pepys, 4.137.

The Sorrowful Bride; or, the London Lasses Lamentation for Her Husbands Insufficiency. London: Printed for R. Kell, 1687. EBBA ID: 21258, Magdalene College Pepys, 3.244.

A True Narrative of the Proceedings at the Sessions-House in the Old-Bayley, at a Sessions There Held on the 1st and 2nd of June, 1677. London: Printed for D.M., 1677.

Allestree, Richard. *The Art of Patience and Balm of Gilead Under All Afflictions an Appendix to the Art of Contentment*. London: Printed by R. Smith for E. Mory, 1694.

Bale, John. *The Actes of Englysh Votaryes Comprehendynge Their Vnchast Practyses*. Antwerp: By S. Mierdman, 1546.

Baley, Walter. *A Briefe Discours of Certain Bathes or Medicinall Waters in the Countie of Warwicke*. London: s.n, 1587.

Barret, Robert. *A Companion for Midwives, Child-Bearing Women, and Nurses Directing Them How to Perform Their Respective Offices*. London: Printed for Thomas Ax, 1699.

Barrin, Jean. *The Monk Unvail'd: Or, a Facetious Dialogue, Discovering the Several Intrigues, and Subtil Practises, Together with the Lewd and Scandalous Lives of Monks, Fryers, and Other Pretended Religious Votaries of the Church of Rome*. London: Printed for Jonathan Edwin, 1678.

Barrough, Philip. *The Methode of Phisicke Conteyning the Causes, Signes, and Cures of Invvard Diseases in Mans Body*. Imprinted at London: By Thomas Vautroullier, 1583.

Basset, Robert. *Curiosities: Or the Cabinet of Nature*. London: Printed by N. and I. Okes, 1637.

Bentley, Thomas. *The Monument of Matrones: Conteining Seuen Seuerall Lamps of Virginitie.* London: H. Denham, 1582.
Boorde, Andrew. *The Breuiary of Healthe, for All Maner of Sicknesses and Diseases.* London: Wyllyam Powell, 1552.
Bradstreet, Anne. *The Works of Anne Bradstreet in Prose and Verse.* Charleston, NC: A.E. Cutter, 1867.
Bunworth, Richard. *The Doctresse.* London: Printed by J.F. for Nicolas Bourne, 1656.
Cavendish, Margaret. *CCXI Sociable Letters Written by the Thrice Noble, Illustrious, and Excellent Princess, the Lady Marchioness of Newcastle.* London: Printed by William Wilson, 1664.
Cavendish, Margaret. *Poems, and Fancies Written by the Right Honourable, the Lady Margaret Newcastle.* London: Printed by T.R. for J. Martin, and J. Allestrye, 1653.
Charles II. *The Letters, Speeches, and Declarations of Charles II.* New York: Funk & Wagnalls, 1968.
Coles, William. *The Art of Simpling. An Introduction to the Knovvledge and Gathering of Plants.* London: Printed by J.G. for Nathaniel Brook, 1656.
Crooke, Helkiah. *Mikrokosmographia a Description of the Body of Man.* London: Printed by William Iaggard, 1615.
Culpeper, Nicholas. *Directory for Midwives.* London: s.n., 1671.
Culpeper, Nicholas. *A Directory for Midwives: or, a Guide for Women, in Their Conception, Bearing, and Suckling Their Children.* London: Printed by Peter Cole, 1651.
Culpeper, Nicholas. *Pharmacopoeia Londinensis, or, the London Dispensatory.* London: Printed by Peter Cole, 1659.
Derham, Samuel. *Hydrologia Philosophica.* Oxford: Printed by Leon. Lichfield for John Howell, 1685.
Drage, William. *Daimonomageia: A Small Treatise of Sicknesses and Diseases from Witchcraft, and Supernatural Causes.* London: Printed by J. Dover, 1665.
Eliot, John. *Poems, or, Epigrams, Satyrs, Elegies, Songs and Sonnets, Upon Several Persons and Occasions.* London: Printed for Henry Brome, 1658.
Fleetwood, William. *The Life and Miracles of St. Wenefride.* London: Printed for S. Buckley, 1713.
Fonteyn, Nicolaas. *The Womans Doctour, or an Exact and Distinct Explanation of All Such Diseases as Are Peculiar to That Sex.* London: Printed for John Blague and Samuel Howes, 1652.
Gibbon, Charles. *A Vvork Vvorth the Reading.* London: Imprinted by Thomas Orwin, 1591.
Gildon, Charles, and John Dunton. *The Post-Boy Rob'd of His Mail, or, the Pacquet Broke Open Consisting of Five Hundred Letters to Persons of Several Qualities*

and Conditions, with Observations Upon Each Letter. London: Printed for John Dunton, 1692.

Gouge, William. *Of Domesticall Duties*. London: Printed by Iohn Haviland for William Bladen, 1622.

Green, Mary Anne Everett. *Letters of Queen Henrietta Maria, Including Her Private Correspondence with Charles I*. London: Richard Bentley, 1857.

Grindal, Edmund. *A Sermon, at the Funeral Solemnitie of the Most High and Mighty Prince Ferdinandus*. London: By Iohn Day, 1564.

Guidott, Thomas. *The Register of Bath or Two Hundred Observations Containing an Account of Cures Performed and Benefit Received by the Use of the Hot Waters of Bath*. London: Printed for Henry Hammond, 1694.

Guillemeau, Jacques. *Child-Birth or, the Happy Deliuerie of Vvomen*. London: Printed by A. Hatfield, 1612.

Hacket, John. *A Century of Sermons Upon Several Remarkable Subjects Preached by the Right Reverend Father in God, John Hacket*. London: Printed by Andrew Clark for Robert Scott, 1675.

Haile, M. *Queen Mary of Modena: Her Life and Letters*. New York: Dent, 1905.

Halkett, Anne. *The Memoirs of Anne, Lady Halkett and Ann, Lady Fanshawe*. Oxford: Clarendon Press, 1979.

Harris, Joseph, and John Webster. *The City Bride, or, the Merry Cuckold*. London: Printed for A. Roper and E. Wilkinson and R. Clavel, 1696.

Harvey, William. *Anatomical Exercitations Concerning the Generation of Living Creatures*. London: Printed by James Young for Octavian Pulleyn, 1653.

Heylyn, Peter. *Cosmographie in Four Bookes*. London: Printed for Henry Seile, 1652.

Hieron, Samuel. *A Helpe Vnto Deuotion*. London: Printed by H. Lownes for Samuell Macham, 1611.

Hippocrates. *The Aphorisms of Hippocrates: With a Translation into Latin and English*. London: A. J. Valpy, 1822.

Holden, Mary. *The Womens Almanack for the Year of Our Lord 1688*. London: Printed by J. Millet, 1688.

Johnson, Edward. *Johnson's Wonder-Working Providence 1628–1651*. New York: Scribner, 1910.

Johnson, Robert. *Enchiridion Medicum, or, a Manual of Physick*. London: Printed by J. Heptinstall for Brabazon Aylmer, 1684.

Jones, John. *The Benefit of the Auncient Bathes of Buckstones*. London: William Iones, 1572.

Lacy, John. *The Dumb Lady, or, the Farriar Made Physician*. London: Printed for Thomas Dring, 1672.

Landi, Ortensio, and Alain Chartier. *Delectable Demaundes, and Pleasaunt Questions, with Their Seuerall Aunswers*. Edited by William Painter. London: By Iohn Cawood for Nicholas Englande, 1566.

The Lisle Letters, ed. Muriel St Clair, Vol. 3 and Vol. 4. Chicago: University of Chicago Press, 1981.

Lupton, Donald. *Obiectorum Reductio: Or, Daily Imployment for the Soule.* London: Printed by Iohn Norton, for Iohn Rothwell, 1634.

Marsh, A. *The Ten Pleasures of Marriage Relating All the Delights and Contentments That Are Mask'd Under the Bands of Matrimony.* London: s.n., 1682.

Massaria, Alessandro, and Robert Turner. *De Morbis Foemineis, the Womans Counsellour: Or, the Feminine Physitian.* London: Printed for John Streater, 1657.

Massaria, Alexander. *Prælectiones De Morbis Mulierum, Conceptus Et Partus*: Lipsiæ, 1600.

Mather, Cotton. *Ornaments for the Daughters of Zion, or, the Character and Happiness of a Vertuous Woman.* Cambridge, MA: Printed by S.G. and B.G. for Samuel Phillips, 1692.

Mauriceau, François. *The Diseases of Women with Child and in Child-Bed*, 2nd ed. London: Printed by John Darby, 1683.

Mordaunt, Elizabeth. *The Priuate Diarie of Elizabeth, Viscountess Mordaunt.* Duncairn: Privately printed, 1856.

Pepys, Samuel. *The Diary of Samuel Pepys, Volume 1.* London: Harper Collins, 1995.

Pepys, Samuel. *The Diary of Samuel Pepys, Volume 3.* London: Harper Collins, 1995.

Pepys, Samuel. *The Diary of Samuel Pepys, Volume 4.* London: Harper Collins, 2000.

Pepys, Samuel. *The Diary of Samuel Pepys, Volume 5.* London: Harper Collins, 2000.

Public Record Office of Great Britain. *CSPVen.* Vol. 20. London: HMSO, 1864.

Raynalde, Thomas, and Eucharius Rösslin. *The Byrth of Mankynde, Otherwyse Named the Womans Booke.* London: By Thomas Raynalde, 1545.

Rivière, Lazare. *The Practice of Physick in Seventeen Several Books*, London: Printed by Peter Cole, 1655.

Robertson, James Craigie. *Materials for the History of Thomas Becket, Archbishop of Canterbury.* London: Longman, 1875.

Robertson, W.H. *A Hand-Book to the Peak of Derbyshire, and to the Use of the Buxton Mineral Waters.* London: Bradbury & Evans, 1854.

Roeslin, Eucharius. *The Byrth of Mankynde, Newly Translated out of Laten into Englysshe.* London: By Thomas Raynalde, 1540.

Rueff, Jakob. 'Book 6'. In *The Expert Midwife, or an Excellent and Most Necessary Treatise of the Generation and Birth of Man.* London: Printed by E. Griffin for S. Burton, 1637.

Salmon, William. *The Family-Dictionary, or, Household Companion.* London: Printed for H. Rhodes, 1696.

Savile, George. *The Lady's New-Years Gift, or, Advice to a Daughter*. London: Printed by Randal Taylor, 1688.

Sharp, Jane. *The Midwives Book, or, the Whole Art of Midwifry Discovered*. London: Printed for Simon Miller, 1671.

Sir Hans Sloane's Correspondence Online. http://drc.usask.ca/projects/sloaneletters/doku.php.

Stanhope, Michael. *Cures Vvithout Care*. London: Printed by William Iones, 1632.

Sudell, Nicholas. *Mulierum Amicus: Or, the Womans Friend*. London: Printed for the author, and is to be sold by J. Hancock in Popes-head-Alley, 1666.

Swift, Jonathan. *The Works of Jonathan Swift*. Edinburgh: Archibald Constable and Co., 1814.

Trotula. *Medieval Woman's Guide to Health: The First English Gynecological Handbook*. Kent, OH: Kent State University Press, 1981.

Trye, Mary. *Medicatrix, or, the Woman-Physician*. London: Printed by T.R. & N. T, 1675.

Whitelocke, Bulstrode. *The Diary of Bulstrode Whitelocke 1605–1675*. Oxford: Oxford University Press, 1990.

Whitelocke, R.H. *Memoirs, Biographical and Historical of Bulstrode Whitelocke, Lord Commissioner of the Great Seal*, London: Routlege, Warne and Routlege, 1860.

Winthrop, John. *The Journal of John Winthrop, 1630–1649*, Vol. 1. Cambridge, MA: Harvard University Press, 1996.

Winthrop, John. *A Short Story of the Rise, Reign, and Ruin of the Antinomians, Familists, and Libertines*. London: Printed for Tho. Parkhurst, 1692.

Wolveridge, James. *Speculum Matricis Hybernicum, or, the Irish Midwives Handmaid*. London: Printed by E. Okes, 1670.

Wright, Abraham. *A Practical Commentary or Exposition Upon the Pentateuch*. London: Printed by G. Dawson, for Tho. Johnson, 1662.

Secondary Literature

The Antinomian Controversy 1636–8: A Documentary History. Middletown, CT: Wesleyan University Press, 1968.

County Court Records of Accomack-Northampton, Virginia, 1632–1640. Washington, DC: American Historical Association, 1954.

Flesh and Spirit: An Anthology of Seventeenth-Century Women's Writing. Manchester: Manchester University Press, 2014.

Seventeenth-Century English Recipe Books: Cooking, Physic and Chirurgery in the Works of Elizabeth Talbot Grey and Aletheia Talbot Howard. Aldershot: Ashgate, 2008.

Adair, Richard. *Courtship, Illegitimacy and Marriage in Early Modern England*. Manchester: Manchester University Press, 1996.

Altbauer-Rudnik, Michal. 'Love Madness and Social Order: Love Melancholy in France and England in the Late Sixteenth and Early Seventeenth Centuries'. *Gesnerus* 63, no. 1/2 (2006): 33–45.

Amussen, Susan Dwyer. *An Ordered Society: Gender and Class in Early Modern England*. New York: Blackwell, 1988.

Anderson, Virginia DeJohn. *New England's Generation: The Great Migration and the Formation of Society and Culture in the Seventeenth Century*. Cambridge: Cambridge University Press, 1991.

Archer, Jayne Elisabeth. 'Women and Chymistry in Early Modern England: The Manuscript Receipt Book (c. 1616) of Sarah Wigges'. In *Gender and Scientific Discourse in Early Modern Culture*, edited by Kathleen P. Long, 191–216. Farnham: Ashgate, 2010.

Barton, Margaret. *Tunbridge Wells*. London: Faber & Faber, 1937.

Bayman, Anna. '"Large Hands, Wide Eares, and Piercing Sights": "The Discoveries" of the Elizabethan and Jacobean Witch Pamphlets'. *Literature & History* 16, no. 1 (2007): 26–45.

Berry, Helen. *The Castrato and His Wife*. Oxford: Oxford University Press, 2011.

Berry, Helen, and Elizabeth A. Foyster. 'Childless Men in Early Modern England'. In *The Family in Early Modern England*, edited by Helen Berry and Elizabeth A. Foyster, 158–183. Cambridge: Cambridge University Press, 2007.

Blair, John. *St Frideswide's Monastery at Oxford: Archaeological and Architectural Studies*. Gloucester: Alan Sutton, 1990.

Blodgett, Harriet. 'Savage, Sarah (1664–1752)'. In *Oxford Dictionary of National Biography, Online ed.*, edited by Lawrence Goldman. Oxford: Oxford University Press, 2004.

Bondeson, J., and A. Molenkamp. 'The Countess Margaret of Henneberg and Her 365 Children'. *Journal of the Royal Society of Medicine* 89, no. 12 (1996): 711–716.

Bono, James Joseph. *The Word of God and the Languages of Man: Interpreting Nature in Early Modern Science and Medicine*. Wisconsin: University of Wisconsin Press, 1995.

Borsay, Peter. *A History of Leisure: The British Experience since 1500*. Basingstoke: Palgrave Macmillan, 2006.

Borsay, Peter. *The Image of Georgian Bath, 1700–2000: Towns, Heritage, and History*. Oxford: Oxford University Press, 2000.

Bowerbank, Sylvia Lorraine, and Sara Heller Mendelson. *Paper Bodies: A Margaret Cavendish Reader*. Peterborough, ON: Broadview Press, 2000.

Bowler, Clara Ann. 'Carted Whores and White Shrouded Apologies: Slander in the County Courts of Seventeenth-Century Virginia'. *The Virginia Magazine of History and Biography* 85, no. 4 (1977): 411–426.

Breitenberg, Mark. *Anxious Masculinity in Early Modern England*. Cambridge: Cambridge University Press, 1996.

Bullough, Vern L. 'An Early American Sex Manual, or, Aristotle Who?'. *Early American Literature* 7, no. 3 (1973): 236–246.

Capp, Bernard. *When Gossips Meet: Women, Family, and Neighbourhood in Early Modern England*. Oxford: Oxford University Press, 2003.

Charlton, Kenneth. *Women, Religion and Education in Early Modern England*. London: Routledge, 2002.

Chaytor, Miranda. 'Household and Kinship: Ryton in the Late 16th and Early 17th Centuries'. *History Workshop* 10 no. 1 (1980): 25–60.

Churchill, Wendy D. *Female Patients in Early Modern Britain: Gender, Diagnosis, and Treatment*. Farnham: Ashgate, 2012.

Cook, Harold John. *The Decline of the Old Medical Regime in Stuart London*. Ithaca, NY: Cornell University Press, 1986.

Cook, Harold John. 'Good Advice and Little Medicine: The Professional Authority of Early Modern English Physicians'. *Journal of British Studies* 33, no. 1 (1994): 1–31.

Cottret, Bernard. *The Huguenots in England: Immigration and Settlement, c. 1550–1700*. Cambridge: Cambridge University Press, 1991.

Crawford, Julie. *Marvelous Protestantism: Monstrous Births in Post-Reformation England*. Baltimore, MD: Johns Hopkins University Press, 2005.

Crawford, Julie. *Mediatrix: Women, Politics*, and *Literary Production in Early Modern England*. Oxford: Oxford University Press, 2014.

Crawford, Patricia. 'Attitudes to Menstruation in Seventeenth-Century England'. *Past & Present* 91 no. 1 (1981): 47–73.

Crawford, Patricia. 'Attitudes to Pregnancy from a Woman's Spiritual Diary, 1687–8'. *Local Population Studies* 21, (1978): 43–45.

Crawford, Patricia. *Blood, Bodies, and Families in Early Modern England*. Harlow: Pearson/Longman, 2004.

Crawford, Patricia. 'Katherine and Philip Henry and Their Children: A Case Study in Family Ideology'. *Transactions of the Historical Society of Lancashire and Cheshire* 134, (1984): 39–73.

Crawford, Patricia. *Women* and *Religion in England 1500–1720*. New York: Routledge, 1993.

Cressy, David. *Birth, Marriage, and Death: Ritual, Religion, and the Life-Cycle in Tudor and Stuart England*. Oxford: Oxford University Press, 1997.

Cressy, David. *Bonfires & Bells: National Memory and the Protestant Calendar in Elizabethan and Stuart England*. Berkeley: University of California Press, 1989.

Cressy, David. *Travesties and Transgressions in Tudor and Stuart England: Tales of Discord and Dissension*. Oxford: Oxford University Press, 2000.

Cross, Claire. 'Hastings, Katherine, Countess of Huntingdon (c.1538–1620)'. In *Oxford Dictionary of National Biography, Online ed.*, edited by Lawrence Goldman. Oxford: Oxford University Press, 2004.

Daston, Lorraine. 'Marvelous Facts and Miraculous Evidence in Early Modern Europe'. *Critical Inquiry* 18, no. 1 (1991): 93–124.

Davies, Owen. *Popular Magic: Cunning Folk in English History*. London: Hambledon Continuum, 2007.

Davis, Natalie Zemon. *The Return of Martin Guerre*. Cambridge, MA: Harvard University Press, 1983.

Dolan, Frances Elizabeth. *Whores of Babylon: Catholicism, Gender, and Seventeenth-Century Print Culture*. Ithaca, NY: Cornell University Press, 1999.

Eccles, Audrey. *Obstetrics and Gynaecology in Tudor and Stuart England*. Kent, OH: Kent State University Press, 1982.

Evans, Jennifer. *Aphrodisiacs, Fertility and Medicine in Early Modern England*. London: Royal Historical Society, 2014.

Evans, Jennifer. '"The Doctor's Wife, (by the Blessing of God) Helps Barrenness": Gender and Infertility Treatments in Early Modern England'. Accepted for publication in *Gender, Health and Medicine in Historical Perspective (Provisional Title)*, edited by Sarah Toulalan.

Evans, Jennifer. 'Female Barrenness, Bodily Access and Aromatic Treatments in Seventeenth-Century England'. *Historical Research* 87, no. 237 (2014): 423–443.

Evans, Jennifer. '"Gentle Purges Corrected with Hot Spices, Whether They Work or Not, Do Vehemently Provoke Venery": Menstrual Provocation and Procreation in Early Modern England'. *Social History of Medicine* 25, no. 1 (2011): 2–19.

Evans, Jennifer. '"They Are Called Imperfect Men": Male Infertility and Sexual Health in Early Modern England'. *Social History of Medicine* 29, no. 2 (2014): 311–332.

Evenden, Doreen. *The Midwives of Seventeenth-Century London*. Cambridge: Cambridge University Press, 1999.

Evenden, Doreen. *Popular Medicine in Seventeenth-Century England*. Bowling Green, OH: Bowling Green State University Popular Press, 1988.

Ewen, Cecil Henry L'Estrange. *Witchcraft and Demonianism: A Concise Account Derived from Sworn Depositions and Confessions Obtained in the Courts of England and Wale*. London: Muller, 1970.

Feinstein-Johnson, Kelly. 'Reading Images and Texts: English Broadside Ballads and Visual Culture, 1600–1800'. Thesis, University of California, Santa Cruz, 2012.

Finucane, Ronald C. *Miracles and Pilgrims: Popular Beliefs in Medieval England*. Totowa, NJ: Rowman and Littlefield, 1977.

Firth, J.B., and N. Erichsen. *Highways and Byways in Derbyshire*. London: Macmillan, 1905.

Fissell, Mary. 'Gender and Generation: Representing Reproduction in Early Modern England'. *Gender & History* 7, no. 3 (1995): 433–456.

Fissell, Mary. 'Hairy Women and Naked Truths: Gender and the Politics of Knowledge in "Aristotle's Masterpiece"'. *William and Mary Quarterly* 60, no. 1 (2003): 43–74.

Fissell, Mary. 'Making a Masterpiece: The Aristotle Texts in Vernacular Medical Culture'. In *Right Living: An Anglo-American Tradition of Self-Help Medicine and Hygiene*, edited by C.E. Rosenberg, 59–88. Baltimore, MD: Johns Hopkins University Press, 2003.

Fissell, Mary. 'The Politics of Reproduction in the English Reformation.'. *Representations* 87, no. 1 (2004): 43–81.

Fissell, Mary. *Vernacular Bodies: The Politics of Reproduction in Early Modern England*. Oxford: Oxford University Press, 2004.

Fitzmaurice, James. 'Cavendish, Margaret, Duchess of Newcastle upon Tyne (1623–1673)'. In *Oxford Dictionary of National Biography, Online ed.*, edited by David Cannadine. Oxford: Oxford University Press, 2004.

Fletcher, Anthony. *Gender, Sex, and Subordination in England, 1500–1800*. New Haven, CT: Yale University Press, 1995.

Fletcher, Anthony. 'The Protestant Idea of Marriage in Early Modern England'. In *Religion, Culture, and Society in Early Modern Britain: Essays in Honour of Patrick Collinson*, edited by Patrick Collinson, Anthony Fletcher and Peter Roberts, xx, 372 p. Cambridge: Cambridge University Press, 1994.

Foster, Thomas A. 'Deficient Husbands: Manhood, Sexual Incapacity, and Male Marital Sexuality in Seventeenth-Century New England'. *The William and Mary Quarterly* 56, no. 4 (1999): 723–744.

Foyster, Elizabeth A. *Manhood in Early Modern England: Honour, Sex, and Marriage*. London: Longman, 1999.

Fraser, Antonia. *The Weaker Vessel*. New York: Knopf, 1984.

Fumerton, Patricia, Anita Guerrini and Kris McAbee. *Ballads and Broadsides in Britain, 1500–1800*. Farnham: Ashgate, 2010.

Furdell, Elizabeth Lane. *Publishing and Medicine in Early Modern England*. Rochester: University of Rochester Press, 2002.

Gélis, Jacques. *History of Childbirth: Fertility, Pregnancy and Birth in Early Modern Europe*. Boston, MA: Rosemary Morris, 1991.

Gibson, Gail McMurray. 'Saint Anne and the Religion of Childbed: Some East Anglian Texts and Talismans'. In *Interpreting Cultural Symbols: Saint Anne in Late Medieval Society*, edited by Kathleen M. Ashley and Pamela Sheingorn, 243 p. Athens: University of Georgia Press, 1990.

Gimbutas, Marija. *The Goddesses and Gods of Old Europe, 6500–3500 BC, Myths and Cult Images*. Berkeley: University of California, 1982.

Goody, Jack. *The Development of the Family and Marriage in Europe*. Cambridge: Cambridge University Press, 1983.

Goose, Nigel, and Liên Luu. *Immigrants in Tudor and Early Stuart England*. Brighton: Sussex Academic Press, 2005.

Gowing, Laura. *Common Bodies: Women, Touch and Power in Seventeenth-Century England*. New Haven, CT: Yale University Press, 2003.

Gowing, Laura. *Gender Relations in Early Modern England*. Harlow: Pearson Education, 2012.

Gowing, Laura. 'Secret Births and Infanticide in Seventeenth-Century England'. *Past & Present* 156, no. 2 (1997): 87–115.

Gray, Todd. *Devon Household Accounts, 1627–59: Henry, Fifth Earl of Bath, and Rachel, Countess of Bath, of Tawstock and London, 1637–1655*. Exeter: Devon and Cornwall Record Society, 1996.

Green, Monica Helen. *Making Women's Medicine Masculine: The Rise of Male Authority in Pre-Modern Gynaecology*. Oxford: Oxford University Press, 2008.

Gregg, Edward. 'Anne (1665–1714)'. In *Oxford Dictionary of National Biography, Online ed.*, edited by Lawrence Goldman. Oxford: Oxford University Press, 2004.

Grummit, David. 'Plantagenet, Arthur, Viscount Lisle (B. Before 1472, D. 1542)'. In *Oxford Dictionary of National Biography, Online ed.*, edited by Lawrence Goldman. Oxford: Oxford University Press, 2004.

Haigh, Christopher. 'The Continuity of Catholicism in the English Reformation'. *Past & Present* 93, no. 1 (1981): 37–69.

Hair, Paul. *Before the Bawdy Court: Selections from Church Court and Other Records Relating to the Correction of Moral Offences in England, Scotland and New England, 1300–1800*. London: Paul Elek, 1972.

Halasz, Alexandra. *The Marketplace of Print: Pamphlets and the Public Sphere in Early Modern England*. Cambridge: Cambridge University Press, 2006.

Hamilton, Anthony. *Memoirs of the Comte De Gramont*. London: Folio Society, 1965.

Hannay, Margaret P. 'Mary Sidney's Other Brothers'. In *Sibling Relations and Gender in the Early Modern World: Sisters, Brothers and Others*, edited by Naomi J. Miller and Naomi Yavneh, 89–103. Aldershot: Ashgate, 2006.

Hannay, Margaret P., Michael G. Brennan and Mary Ellen Lamb. *The Ashgate Research Companion to the Sidneys, 1500–1700: Volume 1: Lives*. Aldershot: Ashgate, 2015.

Harley, David. 'Spiritual Physic, Providence and English Medicine, 1560–1640'. In *Medicine and the Reformation*, edited by Ole Peter Grell and Andrew Cunningham, 101–118. London; New York: Routledge, 1993.

Harris, Tim. *Revolution: The Great Crisis of the British Monarchy, 1685–1720*. London: Allen Lane, 2006.

Harvey, Karen. 'The History of Masculinity, Circa 1650–1800'. *The Journal of British Studies* 44, no. 2 (2005): 296–311.

Heller, Jennifer. *The Mother's Legacy in Early Modern England*. Farnham: Ashgate, 2013.

Hoby, Margaret. *The Private Life of an Elizabethan Lady: The Diary of Lady Margaret Hoby, 1599–1605*. Stroud: Sutton, 1998.

Hsia, Ronnie Po-chia. *The World of Catholic Renewal, 1540–1770*. Cambridge: Cambridge University Press, 1998.

Huard, Leo Albert. 'The Law of Adoption: Ancient and Modern'. *Vanderbilt Law Review* 9, (1955): 743–763.

Hufton, Olwen H. *The Prospect before Her: A History of Women in Western Europe.* New York: Alfred Knopf, 1996.

Hutchinson, Robert. *Thomas Cromwell: The Rise and Fall of Henry VIII's Most Notorious Minister.* New York: Thomas Dunne Books, 2009.

Ingram, Martin. 'Ridings, Rough Music and the "Reform of Popular Culture" in Early Modern England'. *Past & Present* 105, no. 1 (1984): 79–113.

Karlsen, Carol F. *The Devil in the Shape of a Woman: Witchcraft in Colonial New England.* New York: Norton, 1998.

Kassell, Lauren. *Medicine and Magic in Elizabethan London: Simon Forman: Astrologer, Alchemist, and Physician.* Oxford: Oxford University Press, 2007

Keller, Eve. 'The Subject of Touch: Medical Authority in Early Modern Midwifery'. In *Sensible Flesh: On Touch in Early Modern Culture*, edited by E. D. Harvey, 62–80. Philadelphia: University of Pennsylvania Press, 2003.

Kennedy, Gwynne. *Just Anger: Representing Women's Anger in Early Modern England.* Bloomington: South Indiana University Press, 2000.

King, Helen. *Midwifery, Obstetrics and the Rise of Gynaecology: The Uses of a Sixteenth-Century Compendium.* Aldershot: Ashgate, 2007.

Klotz, Edith L. 'A Subject Analysis of English Imprints for Every Tenth Year from 1480 to 1640'. *Huntington Library Quarterly* 1, no. 4 (1938): 417–419.

Knighton, C.S. 'Pepys, Samuel (1633–1703)'. In *Oxford Dictionary of National Biography, Online ed.*, edited by Lawrence Goldman. Oxford: Oxford University Press, 2004.

Koehler, Lyle. 'The Case of the American Jezebels: Anne Hutchinson and Female Agitation During the Years of Antinomian Turmoil, 1636–1640'. *The William and Mary Quarterly* 31, no. 1 (1974): 55–78.

Kouffman, Avra. 'Maternity and Child Loss in Stuart Women's Diaries'. In *Performing Maternity in Early Modern England*, edited by Kathryn M. Moncrief and Kathryn Read McPherson, 171–182. Aldershot: Ashgate, 2007.

Lake, Peter, and Michael C. Questier. *The Antichrist's Lewd Hat: Protestants, Papists and Players in Post-Reformation England.* New Haven, CT: Yale University Press, 2002.

Lang, Amy Schrager. *Prophetic Woman: Anne Hutchinson and the Problem of Dissent in the Literature of New England.* Berkeley: University of California Press, 1989, 1987.

Laqueur, Thomas Walter. *Making Sex: Body and Gender from the Greeks to Freud.* Cambridge, MA: Harvard University Press, 1990.

Larminie, Vivienne. 'Hieron, Samuel (Bap. 1572, D. 1617)'. In *Oxford Dictionary of National Biography, Online ed.*, edited by Lawrence Goldman. Oxford: Oxford University Press, 2004.

Leong, Elaine. '"Herbals She Peruseth": Reading Medicine in Early Modern England'. *Renaissance Studies* 28, no. 4 (2014): 556–578.

Leong, Elaine. 'Making Medicines in the Early Modern Household'. *Bulletin of the History of Medicine* 82, no. 1 (2008): 145–168.

Leong, Elaine, and Sara Pennell. 'Recipe Collections and the Currency of Medical Knowledge in the Early Modern "Medical Marketplace"'. In *Medicine and the Market in England and Its Colonies, c.1450–c.1850*, edited by Mark S.R. Jenner and Patrick Wallis, 133–152. Basingstoke: Palgrave Macmillan, 2007.

Levack, Brian P. *The Witch-Hunt in Early Modern Europe*. London: Longman, 1989.

Lindemann, Mary. *Medicine and Society in Early Modern Europe*. Cambridge: Cambridge University Press, 2010.

Lord, Alexandra M. '"The Great Arcana of the Deity": Menstruation and Menstrual Disorders in Eighteenth-Century British Medical Thought'. *Bulletin of the History of Medicine* 73, no. 1 (1999): 38–63.

MacCarthy, Bridget. *The Female Pen: Women Writers and Novelists, 1621–1818*. New York: NYU Press, 1946.

Macfarlane, Alan. 'Illegitimacy and Illegitimates in English History'. In *Bastardy and Its Comparative History: Studies in the History of Illegitimacy and Marital Nonconformism in Britain, France, Germany, Sweden, North America, Jamaica, and Japan*, edited by Peter Laslett, Karla Oosterveen and Richard Michael Smith, 71–85. Cambridge, MA: Harvard University Press, 1980.

Macfarlane, Alan. *Marriage and Love in England: Modes of Reproduction 1300–1840*. Oxford: Blackwell, 1986.

Maclean, Ian. 'Evidence, Logic, the Rule and the Exception in Renaissance Law and Medicine'. *Early Science and Medicine* 5, no. 3 (2000): 227–257.

Manco, Jean. 'The Cross Bath'. *Bath History* 2, (1988): 49–84.

Matthews-Grieco, Sara F., ed. *Cuckoldry, Impotence and Adultery in Europe*. Aldershot: Ashgate, 2014.

Mayr-Harting, Henry. 'Functions of a Twelfth-Century Shrine: The Miracles of St Frideswide'. In *Studies in Medieval History Presented to R.H.C. Davis*, edited by Henry Mayr-Harting and R. I. Moore, 193–206. London: Hambledon Press, 1985.

McCarl, Mary Rhinelander. 'Publishing the Works of Nicholas Culpeper, Astrological Herbalist and Translator of Latin Medical Works in Seventeenth-Century London'. *Canadian Bulletin of Medical History* 13, no. 2 (1996): 225–276.

McCauliff, C.M.A. 'The First English Adoption Law and Its American Precursors'. *Seton Hall Law Review* 16 (1986): 656.

McClive, Cathy. 'The Hidden Truths of the Belly: The Uncertainties of Pregnancy in Early Modern Europe'. *Social History of Medicine* 15, no. 2 (2002): 209–227.

McClive, Cathy. 'Menstrual Knowledge and Medical Practice in Early Modern France, c. 1555–1761'. In *Menstruation: A Cultural History*, edited by Andrew Shail and Gillian Howie, 76–89. Basingstoke: Palgrave Macmillan, 2005.

McLaren, Angus. *A History of Contraception: From Antiquity to the Present Day.* Oxford: Blackwell, 1990.

McLaren, Angus. *Impotence: A Cultural History.* Chicago: University of Chicago Press, 2007.

McLaren, Angus. *Reproductive Rituals: The Perception of Fertility in England from the Sixteenth to the Nineteenth Century.* London: Methuen, 1984.

McPherson, Kathryn R. '"My Deare Sister": Sainted Sisterhood in Early Modern England'. In *Sibling Relations and Gender in the Early Modern World: Sisters, Brothers and Others*, edited by Naomi J. Miller and Naomi Yavneh, 182–194. Aldershot: Ashgate, 2006.

McShane, Angela J. *Political Broadside Ballads of Seventeenth-Century England: A Critical Bibliography.* London: Pickering & Chatto, 2011.

Melville, Lewis. *Society at Royal Tunbridge Wells in the Eighteenth Century and After.* London: Nash, 1912.

Mendelson, Sara Heller. *Margaret Cavendish.* Farnham: Ashgate, 2009.

Mendelson, Sara Heller, and Patricia Crawford. *Women in Early Modern England: 1550–1720.* Oxford: Oxford University Press, 1998.

Mendelson, Sara Heller, and Mary O'Connor. '"Thy Passionately Loving Sister and Faithfull Friend": Anne Dormer's Letters to Her Sister Lady Trumbull'. In *Sibling Relations and Gender in the Early Modern World: Sisters, Brothers and Others*, edited by Naomi J. Miller and Naomi Yavneh, xiv, 238 p. Aldershot: Ashgate, 2006.

Morrison, Susan Signe. *Women Pilgrims in Late Medieval England: Private Piety and Public Performance.* London: Routledge, 2000.

Mortimer, Ian. *The Dying and the Doctors: The Medical Revolution in Seventeenth-Century England.* Woodbridge: Boydell & Brewer, 2015.

Muir, Edward. *Ritual in Early Modern Europe.* Cambridge: Cambridge University Press, 1997.

Mullett, Charles F. *Public Baths and Health in England, 16th–18th Century.* Baltimore, MD: The Johns Hopkins Press, 1946.

Newhauser, Richard. '"These Seaven Devils": The Capital Vices on the Way to Modernity'. In *Sin in Medieval and Early Modern Culture: The Tradition of the Seven Deadly Sins*, edited by Richard Newhauser and Susan Janet Ridyard, 157–188. York: York Medieval Press, 2012.

Newton, Hannah. *The Sick Child in Early Modern England, 1580–1720.* Oxford: Oxford University Press, 2012.

O'Brien, Karen. *White Magic and the Cunning Folk: Charms and Blessings in Northwest England.* Liverpool: Bluecoat Press, 2001.

O'Donnell, Mary Ann. *Aphra Behn: An Annotated Bibliography of Primary and Secondary Sources*. Aldershot: Ashgate, 2004.

O'Hara, Diana. *Courtship and Constraint: Rethinking the Making of Marriage in Tudor England*. Manchester: UK Manchester University Press, 2000.

Oren-Magidor, Daphna. 'From Anne to Hannah: Religious Views of Infertility in Post-Reformation England'. *Journal of Women's History* 27, no. 3 (2015): 86–108.

Oren-Magidor, Daphna. 'Literate Laywomen, Male Medical Practitioners and the Treatment of Fertility Problems in Early Modern England'. *Social History of Medicine* 29, no. 2 (2016): 290–310.

Oren-Magidor, Daphna, and Catherine Rider. 'Introduction: Infertility in Medieval and Early Modern Medicine'. *Social History of Medicine* 29, no. 2 (2016): 211–223.

Osborne, Bruce, and Cora Weaver. *Aquae Britannia: Rediscovering 17th Century Springs & Spas*. Malvern: Cora Weaver, 1996.

Park, Katharine. *Secrets of Women: Gender, Generation, and the Origins of Human Dissection*. New York; Cambridge, MA: Zone Books, Distributed by the MIT Press, 2006.

Paster, Gail Kern. *The Body Embarrassed: Drama and the Disciplines of Shame in Early Modern England*. Ithaca, NY: Cornell University Press, 1993.

Pelling, Margaret. *Medical Conflicts in Early Modern London: Patronage, Physicians, and Irregular Practitioners 1550–1640*. Oxford: Oxford University Press, 2003.

Pelling, Margaret. 'Thoroughly Resented? Older Women and the Medical Role in Early Modern London.' In *Women, Science and Medicine, 1500–1700: Mothers and Sisters of the Royal Society*, edited by Lynette Hunter and Sarah Hutton, xx, 292 p. Stroud: Sutton, 1997.

Peters, Christine. 'Gender Sacrament and Ritual: The Making and Meaning of Marriage in Late Medieval and Early Modern England'. *Past & Present* 169, no. 1 (2000): 63–96.

Pincus, Steven. *1688: The First Modern Revolution*. New Haven, CT: Yale University Press, 2009.

Pinto, L.B. 'The Folk Practice of Gynecology and Obstetrics in the Middle Ages'. *Bulletin of the History of Medicine* 47, no. 5 (1973): 513–523.

Pollock, Linda A. 'Childbearing and Female Bonding in Early Modern England'. *Social History* 22, no. 3 (1997): 286–306.

Pollock, Linda A. 'Embarking on a Rough Passage: The Experience of Pregnancy in Early-Modern Society'. In *Women as Mothers in Pre-Industrial England: Essays in Memory of Dorothy McLaren* edited by Valerie A. Fildes and Dorothy McLaren, 39–67. London: Routledge, 1990.

Porter, Dorothy, and Roy Porter. *Patient's Progress: Doctors and Doctoring in Eighteenth- Century England*. Stanford, CA: Stanford University Press, 1989.

Porter, Roy. 'The Patient's View'. *Theory and Society* 14 (1985): 175–198.

Raber, Karen L. '"Our Wits Joined as in Matrimony": Margaret Cavendish's *Playes* and the Drama of Authority'. In *Margaret Cavendish*, edited by Sara Heller Mendelson, 73–102. Farnham: Ashgate, 2009.

Rankin, Alisha. 'Duchess, Heal Thyself: Elisabeth of Rochlitz and the Patient's Perspective in Early Modern Germany'. *Bulletin of the History of Medicine* 82, no. 1 (2008): 109–144.

Rattue, James. *The Living Stream: Holy Wells in Historical Context*. Woodbridge: Boydell Press, 1995.

Reeser, Todd W. *Moderating Masculinity in Early Modern Culture*. Chapel Hill: University of North Carolina Press, 2006.

Rickman, Johanna. *Love, Lust, and License in Early Modern England: Illicit Sex and the Nobility*. Aldershot: Ashgate, 2008.

Rider, Catherine. 'Men and Infertility in Late Medieval English Medicine'. *Social History of Medicine* 29, no. 2 (2016): 245–266

Rochester, John Wilmot. *John Wilmot, Earl of Rochester: The Poems, and Lucina's Rape*. Malden, MA: Wiley-Blackwell, 2010.

Roland Mushat, Frye. 'The Teachings of Classical Puritanism on Conjugal Love'. *Studies in the Renaissance* 2, (1955): 148–159.

Rollins, Hyder E. 'The Three Hundred and Sixty Five Children'. *Notes and Queries* s2-IX, 237 (1922), 351b–353.

Roper, Lyndal. *Oedipus and the Devil: Witchcraft, Sexuality, and Religion in Early Modern Europe*. London; New York: Routledge, 1994.

Roper, Lyndal. *Witch Craze: Terror and Fantasy in Baroque Germany*. New Haven, CT: Yale University Press, 2004.

Rublack, Ulinka. 'Pregnancy Childbirth and the Female Body in Early Modern Germany'. *Past & Present* 150 (1996): 84–110.

Scholz, Susanne. *Body Narratives: Writing the Nation and Fashioning the Subject in Early Modern England*. Basingstoke: Palgrave Macmillan, 2000.

Schwoerer, Lois G. *The Revolution of 1688–89: Changing Perspectives*. Cambridge: Cambridge University Press, 1992.

Searle, Arthur. *Barrington Family Letters 1628–1632*. London: Royal Historical Society, 1983.

Shagan, Ethan H. *The Rule of Moderation: Violence, Religion and the Politics of Restraint in Early Modern England*. Cambridge: Cambridge University Press, 2011.

Sharpe, James. *Defamation and Sexual Slander in Early Modern England: The Church Courts at York*. York: University of York Press, 1980.

Sharpe, James. *English Witchcraft, 1560–1736*. 6 vols. London: Pickering & Chatto, 2003.

Sharpe, James. *Witchcraft in Early Modern England*. Harlow: Longman, 2001.

Shepard, Alexandra. *Meanings of Manhood in Early Modern England*. Oxford: Oxford University Press, 2003.

Shoemaker, Robert Brink. *Gender in English Society, 1650–1850: The Emergence of Separate Spheres?* London: Longman, 1998.

Slater, Miriam. *Family Life in the Seventeenth Century: The Verneys of Claydon House.* London: Routledge, 1984.

Smith, Lisa W. 'Imagining Women's Fertility before Technology'. *Journal of Medical Humanities* 31, no. 1 (2010): 69–79.

Smith, Lisa W. 'La Raillerie Des Femmes? Les Femmes, La Stérilité Et La Société En France a L'époque Moderne. In *Femmes En Fleurs, Femmes En Corps: Sang, Santé, Sexualités Du Moyen Age Aux Lumières*, edited by Cathy McClive and Nicole Pellegrin, 203–220. Saint-Étienne: Publications de l'Université de Saint-Étienne, 2010.

Speck, W.A. 'Mary II (1662–1694)'. In *Oxford Dictionary of National Biography, Online ed.*, edited by Lawrence Goldman. Oxford: Oxford University Press, 2004.

Stone, Lawrence. *The Family, Sex and Marriage in England, 1500–1800.* New York: Harper & Row, 1977.

Symcotts, John. *A Seventeenth Century Doctor and His Patients: John Symcotts, 1592–1662.* Bedfordshire: Bedfordshire Record Society, 1951.

Taavitsainen, Irma, and Päivi Pahta. *Medical Writing in Early Modern English.* Cambridge: Cambridge University Press, 2011.

Tadmor Naomi. 'Early Modern English Kinship in the Long Run: Reflections on Continuity and Change'. *Continuity and Change* 25, no. 1 (2010): 15–48.

Tadmor Naomi. *Family and Friends in Eighteenth-Century England: Household, Kinship and Patronage.* Cambridge: Cambridge University Press, 2001.

Thomas, Keith. *Religion and the Decline of Magic.* New York: Scribner, 1971.

Thomas, Samuel S. 'Early Modern Midwifery: Splitting the Profession, Connecting the History'. *Journal of Social History* 43, no. 1 (2009): 115–138.

Tilley, Morris P. *A Dictionary of Proverbs in England in the 16th and 17th Centuries.* Ann Arbor: University of Michigan Press, 1950.

Toulalan, Sarah. '"Elderly Years Cause a Total Dispaire of Conception": Old Age, Sex and Infertility in Early Modern England'. *Social History of Medicine* 29, no. 2 (2015): 333–359.

Toulalan, Sarah. *Imagining Sex: Pornography and Bodies in Seventeenth-Century England.* Oxford: Oxford University Press, 2007.

Toulalan, Sarah. '"To[O] Much Eating Stifles the Child": Fat Bodies and Reproduction in Early Modern England'. *Historical Research* 87, no. 235 (2014): 65–93.

Trevor-Roper, Hugh. *Europe's Physician: The Various Life of Sir Théodore De Mayerne.* New Haven, CT: Yale University Press, 2006.

Trussell, J., and C. Wilson. 'Sterility in a Population with Natural Fertility'. *Population Studies* 39, no. 2 (1985): 269–286.

Underdown, David E. 'The Taming of the Scold: The Enforcement of Patriarchal Authority in Early Modern England. In *Order and Disorder in Early Modern England*, edited by Anthony J. Fletcher. Cambridge: Cambridge University Press, 1985.

Ungerer, Gustav. 'Roland Du Jardin: Author of a Discourse of the Married and Single Life?'. *The Library* s6-II, no. 2 (1980): 211–216.

Van Dorsten, Jan. *Poets, Patrons and Professors: Sir Philip Sidney, Daniel Rogers and the Leiden Humanists*. Oxford: Oxford University Press, 1962.

Wahrman, Dror. 'Change and the Corporeal in Seventeenth- and Eighteenth Century Gender History: Or, Can Cultural History Be Rigorous?'. *Gender & History* 20, no. 3 (2008): 584–602.

Walsham, Alexandra. 'Holywell, Contesting Sacred Space in Post-Reformation Wales'. In *Sacred Space in Early Modern Europe*, edited by Will Coster and Andrew Spicer, 211–236. Cambridge: Cambridge University Press, 2005.

Walsham, Alexandra. *Providence in Early Modern England*. Oxford: Oxford University Press, 1999.

Waters, Claire M. 'Power and Authority'. In *A Companion to Middle English Hagiography*, edited by Sarah Salih, ix, 182 p. Woodbridge, Rochester, NY: D.S. Brewer, 2006.

Watt, Tessa. *Cheap Print and Popular Piety, 1550–1640*. Cambridge: Cambridge University Press, 1991.

Wear, Andrew. *Knowledge and Practice in English Medicine, 1550–1680*. Cambridge: Cambridge University Press, 2000.

Wear, Andrew. 'Medicine in Early Modern Europe 1500–1700. In *The Western Medical Tradition: 800 BC to AD 1800*, edited by Lawrence I. Conrad, 215–249. Cambridge: Cambridge University Press, 1995.

Wear, Andrew. 'Religious Beliefs and Medicine in Early Modern England'. In *Health and Healing in Early Modern England: Studies in Social and Intellectual History*, edited by Andrew Wear. Aldershot: Ashgate, 1998.

Webb, Diana. *Pilgrimage in Medieval England*. London: Hambledon and London, 2000.

Weber, A.S. 'Women's Early Modern Medical Almanacs in Historical Context'. *English Literary Renaissance* 33, no. 3 (2003): 358–402.

Weil, Rachel. 'The Politics of Legitimacy: Women and the Warming-Pan Scandal. In *The Revolution of 1688–89: Changing Perspectives*, edited by Lois G. Schwoerer, 65–82. Cambridge: Cambridge University Press, 1992.

Westerkamp, Marilyn J. 'Anne Hutchinson, Sectarian Mysticism, and the Puritan Order'. *Church History* 59, no. 4 (1990): 482–496.

Whaley, Leigh. *Women and the Practice of Medical Care in Early Modern Europe, 1400–1800*. Basingstoke: Palgrave Macmillan, 2011.

Wiesner, Merry E. *Christianity and Sexuality in the Early Modern World: Regulating Desire, Reforming Practice*, 2nd ed. London: Routledge, 2010.

Wiesner, Merry E. *Women and Gender in Early Modern Europe*, 2nd ed., Vol. 20. Cambridge: Cambridge University Press, 2000.

Wilson, Adrian. *The Making of Man-Midwifery: Childbirth in England, 1660–1770*. Cambridge, MA: Harvard University Press, 1995.

Wilson, Adrian. *Ritual and Conflict: The Social Relations of Childbirth in Early Modern England*. Farnham: Ashgate, 2016.

Wilson, Derek A. *All the King's Women: Love, Sex and Politics in the Life of Charles II*. London: Hutchinson, 2003.

Winship, Michael P. *The Times and Trials of Anne Hutchinson: Puritans Divided*. Lawrence: University Press of Kansas, 2005.

Wrigley, E.A., R.S. Davies, J.E. Oeppen and R.S. Schofield. *English Population History from Family Reconstitution 1580–1837*. Cambridge: Cambridge University Press, 1997.

INDEX

D. Oren-Magidor, *Infertility in Early Modern England*,
Early Modern History: Society and Culture,
DOI 10.1057/978-1-137-47668-5

CPSIA information can be obtained
at www.ICGtesting.com
Printed in the USA
LVHW07*1033050318
568683LV00008B/25/P

9 781137 476678